7 Days to
Amazing
Sex

7 Days to Amazing Sex

Revolutionise your life and feel sexy now

SARAH HEDLEY

piatkus

PIATKUS

First published in Great Britain in 2010 by Piatkus

A CIP catalogue record for this book is available from the British Library

ISBN 978-0-7499-4090-4

Text designed and set by Sam Charrington Design
Illustrations by Andrew Archer
Cover photographs by Malin Enberg
Printed and bound in Great Britain by CPI Mackays, Chatham ME5 8TD

Papers used by Piatkus are natural, renewable and recyclable products
sourced from well-managed forests and certified in accordance with the
rules of the Forest Stewardship Council.

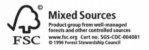

Piatkus
An imprint of
Little, Brown Book Group
100 Victoria Embankment
London EC4Y 0DY

An Hachette UK Company
www.hachette.co.uk
www.piatkus.co.uk

To all the couples that care enough
to make a change

Acknowledgements

With thanks to all the people who have shared their real-life sex confessions (though some names have been changed to protect the guilty, they know who they are); *Scarlet* magazine's previous owner Wesley Stanton, who kindly allowed me to reproduce my favourite erotic fiction stories from the title; my super agent Gordon Wise, who lives up to his name; editor Helen Stanton and all the team at Little, Brown who shared my vision; Alan, Brenda, Wendy, Gordon, Pauline and Bill – my parents, step-parents and in-laws respectively, who all seemed to worry about me hitting my deadline as much as I did; and, of course, to the man who made that happen – my husband Paul – by offering to do all the housework until my book was finished, which, as any woman knows, is one of the best forms of foreplay there is!

Contents

Introduction

Meet Your Tutor

After fifteen years of working as a magazine journalist, specialising in sex, health and well-being, I'm now recognised as one of the UK's leading authorities on these topics. I've resided as sex editor of both *Cosmopolitan* and *Maxim* magazines, and as sex and relationships columnist for the UK's biggest-selling newspaper, the *Sun*. As one of the founding editors of *Scarlet*, I also helped create the first mainstream British women's magazine devoted to delivering the message 'no diets, more sex', and I've contributed to countless other magazines internationally, including *Men's Health, Men's Fitness, FHM, Company, Shape, more!* and *Top Sante*.

In my roles of agony aunt, health expert and social commentator, I've appeared on over a hundred television and radio shows around the world, including *Oprah, Richard & Judy, When Sex Goes Wrong* and *Cosmopolitan's 50 Ways to Please* series. I've also written and co-directed my own sex education DVD series, *Modern Loving*.

In addition, contributions to the world's bookshelves include acting as consulting expert on *The Rough Guide to Men's Health* (Rough Guides) and my first tome of carnal knowledge *Sex by Numbers* (Piatkus), which has been translated into six languages.

What 7 *Days to Amazing Sex* Can Do For You

What if I told you I knew of a special treatment that could make you look ten years younger? What if I told you the same treatment could help you live longer, drop a dress size and defend against serious illness? Would you want to know what it was?

Of course you would; and I wrote this book to tell you – that treatment is sex.

So few people appreciate the influence a healthy sex life can have on their overall mental and physical well-being. After reading *7 Days to Amazing Sex* though, you'll want to have sex more often and you'll have the skills, confidence and techniques to enjoy each and every encounter to the full. As a result, you'll look and feel amazing. But don't just take my word for it – check out what science has shown us.

The Science Bit

- **Look younger.** A study has shown that having sex three times a week or more can make you look ten years younger than the average adult who has sex only twice a week. Dr David Weeks, consultant neuropsychologist at Scotland's Royal Edinburgh Hospital, interviewed 3500 people aged between 18 and 102 in Britain, Europe and the US and found that, 'pleasure derived from sex is a crucial factor in preserving youth'. This is because sex pumps oxygen around the body, delivering essential nutrients to the skin, while hormones released during sex have a positive effect on how we age.

- **Live longer.** Queens University in Northern Ireland monitored 1000 middle-aged men over the course of a decade and discovered a lower death rate among those who had the most orgasms, and that those who had sex three or more times a week reduced their risk of suffering a heart attack or stroke by half.

- **Reduce weight and improve overall fitness.** Sex is a brilliant form of exercise. It's estimated that a vigorous twenty-minute session can burn up to 200 calories; sustaining sexual positions can help improve flexibility and muscle tone; at the same time the pulse can rise from 70 to 150 beats per minute, giving the heart a cardiovascular workout. And, best of all, there are no gym fees.

● **Defend against illness, including prostate cancer and incontinence.** A study by Wilkes University in Pennsylvania, US, showed that people who had sex once or twice a week had 30 per cent higher levels of immunoglobulin A (an antibody that boosts the immune system) than those who abstained.

Over time, prolonged deep kissing has been shown to lower blood pressure and cholesterol levels; in the short-term, kissing releases bacteria that stimulates the production of antibodies, which help fight infection.

The same muscles used during sex are used for bladder control, so regular sexual activity also helps fight stress incontinence, which affects 15 million people – primarily women – around the world.

For men, regular ejaculation has been linked to lower risk of prostate cancer. A study published by the *British Journal of Urology International* said that men in their twenties can reduce their risk of prostate cancer by a third if they ejaculate more than five times a week.

● **Boost self-esteem.** The chemical reaction caused by having sex activates the body's natural opiates, which results in a general feeling of contentment. There has even been some research into the benefits of unprotected sex with an STI-free partner. Prostaglandin – found in semen – is thought to be absorbed by the female body, where it works to balance a woman's hormones and helps alleviate depression.

● **Relieve pain.** In women, oestrogen production increases as a result of sex, which helps combat period pains. In fact, just about everything from arthritis to the humble ('Not tonight dear, I've got a . . . ') headache can be soothed with sex. This is because, just prior to orgasm, levels of the hormone oxytocin increase to release endorphins that act as natural painkillers.

● **Reduce stress.** Ironically, though stress is a major libido-killer, the endorphins released during lovemaking help combat stress – some reports suggest that even holding hands can aid in stress relief.

● **Cure insomnia.** Forget taking over-the-counter drugs – an orgasm has long been known to be an effective, totally safe, quick-fix cure for insomnia.

● **Improve your relationship.** The hormone oxytocin is linked with emotional bonding, and helps boost intimacy between you and your partner to make your relationship a happier one.

Once you appreciate all of the life-changing benefits an exciting and active sex life can bring, you're sure to be ready to follow *7 Days to Amazing Sex*. A sexier new you awaits – all you need to do is turn the page and read on . . .

How to Plan Your Seven Days to Amazing Sex

The Timetable

You will need to invest around two hours per day, but the seven-day plan is extremely flexible: you can follow it over seven consecutive days, at home or even on holiday, or you can fit the days in around your own schedule, whenever suits you best, for example one day a week over seven weeks.

The Rules

All sexual contact between couples is forbidden on Day One; penetrative sex is strictly forbidden until Day Four.

Course Notes and Extra-curricular Activities

Throughout the seven-day plan you will find 'Course Notes' offering useful tips and info to support your sexual studies. You'll also find 'Extra-curricular Activities' to try outside of plan hours.

Course Requirements

You will need pens, paper, massage lotion and lubricant (or a two-in-one massage lubricant), condoms (if you use them) and a selection of sex toys (or household substitutes), details of which will be given on the relevant days of the plan.

7 Days to Amazing Sex has been created in the knowledge that a full and satisfying sex life is one of the keys to overall happiness and well-being, and the aim is not only to deliver that message, but also to make it happen. This is an action-packed sex plan, designed to satisfy every reader – not just for seven days, but for the rest of their lives.

Have fun!

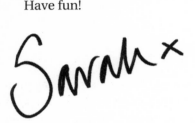

Day One
You Time

In picking up this book, you've let me into your sex life, so now I'm going to let you into mine.

I didn't start masturbating until I was in my twenties. I wasn't a virgin – I'd been living with a long-term boyfriend and we had a healthy sex life, but it was only when I became single again, and my career as a sex writer began, that I started masturbating, primarily as a way to research the techniques I was writing about. Once I started my journey into solo sex – and, boy, what a journey it was! – it dawned on me just how bizarre it was that I hadn't done it sooner. Because I'd always had a boyfriend, I'd solely relied on another person to fulfil all my sexual needs. What pressure that is to put on a relationship, and what a waste of the body I'd been given.

Masturbation is a pure and simple pleasure. It's free, it's fun and it's healthy, and, in my opinion (and that of many medical experts), it's just as good for you as taking a daily multivitamin.

During your first day on my plan I'm going to show you how to take solo sex to a whole new level, even if you're already a proficient self-pleasurer. And if you're not? Don't be shy – you'll be working alone.

Note: sexual interaction of any kind with your partner is strictly forbidden until Day Two of the plan – even outside of programme hours! Right now, your only goal is to enjoy your body alone. All you need are a few hours to spare and some props (more on those later). But first, I'd like to test your knowledge of solo sex . . .

Exercise A

The Solo Sex Quiz – How Much Do You Really Know About Masturbation

Without peeking at the answers, work together with your partner and think about the following questions, then jot down your responses on a piece of paper.

1. What are the benefits of masturbation?

2. How often should a person masturbate?

3. Are your masturbation habits normal?

4. How could they tell Pinocchio was lying?

Answers at the ready? Now check below to see how many you got right, and see whether I can convince you to increase your solo sex indulgences.

Answers

1. What are the benefits of masturbation?

When it comes to self-pleasuring, sex experts all agree that masturbation can lead the way to a much happier and healthier life, in and out of the bedroom. Here's why:

- **It's the safest form of sex there is.** With no risk of STIs or pregnancy, solo sex offers a blissful, worry-free experience. All you need to think about are the sensations.

- **It's good for your health.** Studies show that regular orgasms offer a host of health benefits from reducing stress to defending against major illnesses like prostate cancer.

- **It makes partner sex better.** Maybe you've only ever had partners who have instinctively known which buttons to push without you uttering a word of advice, but let me tell you, you're

Extra-curricular Activity
Mass debate

Despite the benefits, many people in relationships don't masturbate; some feel it's a taboo or an infidelity of sorts, while others say their partner objects to them doing so. If you have objections to your partner masturbating, it's time to talk about it now. Is your opposition founded, or might it be borne of your own low self-esteem? For example, some men feel intimidated by their lover's use of sex toys, and some women feel jealous over a partner's arousal through pornography, or even fantasy. And then there are people who feel disappointed that they're not enough for their partner or who have been told from an early age that it's wrong to masturbate.

Well, it isn't wrong to masturbate – it's rare to have identically matched libidos and a person shouldn't have to deny their solo sexual urges. Often we project our own negativity in situations that make us feel uncomfortable, so we may catch a partner masturbating and accuse them of being disgusting, when really we're angry with ourselves for not being as sexually free as they seem to be. Or we may accuse a lover of being sex mad, when in actual fact we are jealous of their naturally higher libido.

If you have objections to your partner masturbating, take a moment to write down the reasons for them – and be honest with yourself. You don't ever have to show your partner what you've written, but it can be liberating to open up about this, and when your partner knows how you feel, it allows them the opportunity to offer reassurance and compromise. There are almost always solutions to any issues, but you have to start talking in order to find them.

in the minority. For most of us, good sex is the result of intimate knowledge of our own sexual hot spots and an eagerness to communicate that information to our lovers. Learn how to satisfy yourself, and you're already halfway to having a mind-blowing sex life with your partner.

● **It's a libido booster.** Masturbating more often can actually help keep your libido charged. Think of your libido as you would a car – the less you drive it, the more likely the engine is to seize up. For many people, their sex drive works in the same way. So the more sex you have, the more sex you tend to want, and masturbation is a good way to keep your sexual batteries charged.

The benefits of pelvic-floor toning for men

- A 2004 study from the University of Bristol found that pelvic toning can help overcome erectile dysfunction and achieve the same results as Viagra without the associated health risks of taking a drug.

- Studies have shown that pelvic workouts for men can 'increase awareness of sexual sensations and enhance enjoyment'.

- Pelvic-floor exercises are recommended for men following a prostatectomy, and research has shown that pelvic-floor strengthening can improve sexual function and overcome incontinence.

The benefits of pelvic floor toning for women

- Regular pelvic-floor toning helps prevent stress incontinence, a condition that affects many women from as young as their twenties, particularly those who have been through childbirth.

- Pelvic toning increases blood flow to the genitals, which increases sensitivity, making sex more enjoyable.

- Orgasm is a series of muscular contractions; strengthening pelvic muscles will therefore increase the power of orgasms.

- Toning the pelvic muscles tightens the vaginal canal, creating a snugger fit for your partner and making any penis feel bigger.

● **It's a libido balancer.** I often receive letters from people who complain that their partner's libido is higher or lower than their own. This is one of the most common problems couples face. I recommend masturbation as a 'libido balancer' as it works in two ways. Firstly, those with lower libidos can help rev their sex drive by masturbating. Secondly, those with naturally high libidos can self-pleasure to satisfy themselves. Without this outlet for their sexual energies, the lover with the higher libido can place undue pressure, knowingly or otherwise, on their partner. This can lead to resentment and make the partner with the lower libido feel coerced, or even like a sexual failure. When a person's sex drive is already flagging, this can feel like the final nail in the coffin of their libido.

● **It's guaranteed sex for singles.** Develop good solo sex skills and you'll never feel sexually deprived again, regardless of your relationship status. Knowing how to self-pleasure well is empowering, and it will work in your favour when you find yourself back on the dating scene. When you don't need another person to fulfil you, you'll subconsciously give off an air of independence and confidence that others will be naturally drawn to.

Extra-curricular Activity
Sexercise

It's easy to incorporate a pelvic-floor workout into self-pleasuring, because rather than being a chore, it actually enhances sensation for you. Start by drawing blood into your genitals by pumping the pelvic-floor muscles ten times as quickly as you can. Then squeeze and hold the muscles for five seconds, and release. Don't hold your breath as you 'work out' – it improves sensation when you breathe evenly. Repeat this set of exercises three times, focusing on how your genitals feel as they begin to warm up, and on how they're going to feel when you finally touch them (think of it as a form of teasing foreplay for full-on masturbation). Next, as you stimulate yourself, clench and release the pelvic-floor muscles in time to the rhythm of your stroke, and, finally, when you feel your climax approaching, rapidly clench and release the muscles again until orgasm takes over your body.

● **It's the fun way to do your pelvic-floor workout.** For many decades, women have been advised to work their pelvic-floor muscles (also referred to as the pubococcygeal or PC muscles), but it's now understood that it's just as vital for men to exercise this group of muscles, and recommended workout regimes are similar for both men and women.

The pelvic-floor muscles are shaped like a sling and attach to the pubic bone and coccyx (tailbone). They hold the bladder and urethra (the tube that carries urine from the bladder and out of the body) in place. When we urinate, our pelvic-floor muscles relax as the bladder contracts to let out urine. So, you can see why pelvic-muscle strength and incontinence are linked.

To feel your pelvic muscles in action, stop peeing mid-flow – and the muscles will lift and tighten. However, only do this to identify the muscles, as repeatedly interrupting urinary flow can be damaging. When pelvic toning you should focus on these muscles only; the surrounding muscles in your thighs, bottom and stomach should be relaxed.

Doctors recommend using a squeeze- (or lift-) and-release technique to exercise the pelvic floor, gradually building the number of repetitions as you progress. You could start by doing thirty a day and work up from there. You can also vary the pace of repetitions; for example, you could perform ten slow repetitions, followed by five faster ones.

As with all forms of exercise, it can be difficult to find the motivation, but when it comes to pelvic toning, masturbation can *be* that motivation. Try my Sexercise workout (see p.11) later today, or any other time when you're indulging in solo sex, and you'll see what I mean.

Real Sex
Star of the Show

I always fantasise when I masturbate. Most often, I just relive things that have happened between me and my girlfriend in the past – I like to be the star of my own show – though in my fantasies we sometimes go a little further than we have in real life. For example, we'll always have anal sex, which is not something we do in real life, and my girlfriend will always be wearing sexy lingerie.

Michael, 22

2. How often should a person masturbate?

The benefits of regular masturbation have been proven, but there's no such thing as a 'right' number of times to indulge. One survey of over 3000 people showed that a small majority (around 20 per cent) masturbate one to two times a week when in a steady relationship, while others do it every day, some never do, and the rest fall somewhere in between.

Factors that affect how often we masturbate tend to be the same as those that influence how often we have sex, namely: time, opportunity, libido, general health and our personal feelings towards masturbation and our own bodies. When we adopt a positive attitude towards masturbation, we're more likely to masturbate regularly and reap the rewards, which, in turn, motivate us to carry on. Start masturbating today (if you weren't already) and pledge to satisfy your solo sex urges whenever they arise, regardless of whether or not it's convenient – even if it means nipping into the office toilet!

Real Sex
Whirlpool Romance

I've never been a fan of masturbating with a shower head the way a lot of women do, as I find the sensation too mild, but I have tried it in a whirlpool bath before. I was at my local gym one weekday and it was very quiet. The whirlpool bath overlooks the swimming pool and there was one male swimmer, shooting up and down the lanes, not paying me any attention. I hadn't intended to masturbate, but a jet of water caught my clitoris in just the right way, and I instantly felt turned on. I was able to pull my swimsuit to one side and position my clit in a constant stream of water, which made me come in minutes. I didn't fancy the swimmer, but just knowing he was in the same room made me feel extra naughty.

Louise, 31

3. Are your masturbation habits normal?

Some people worry that their masturbation habits are a little odd; they think that the subject matter of their fantasies or the props they use would be perceived to be weird or deviant by others. But just as there's no correct number of times to self-pleasure, there's no set-in-stone etiquette to follow in fantasies either.

In her groundbreaking book *My Secret Garden*, Nancy Friday revealed that women fantasise about everything from rape scenarios to sex with animals. Having these fantasies does not mean that these women actually want to be raped or to dabble in bestiality in real life. In rape fantasies the woman is completely in control, but the fantasy allows her to relinquish the guilt of wanting sex because she's being 'forced' into it. This is possibly why rape fantasies are so common among women who were brought up to believe sex is sinful or dirty. The thrill of fantasising about having sex with animals is more often about breaking a huge taboo and feeling as kinky as possible. The same can be said of people fantasising about sex with their partner's siblings or best friends. Breaking the rules – even in fantasy – can trigger sexual adrenalin.

Real Sex
Swinging Into Action

Myself and my husband would never dream of going to a swingers' party. We're strictly monogamous, and, to be honest, I think the reality of one would scare me, but I've read so many stories about them in magazines that I've visualised how they might be. In my fantasies, I'm openly having sex with my husband at one of these parties and there are men surrounding us, all of them masturbating over the sight of us. As they reach their climaxes, so do I.

Margaret, 47

For men, there's still a great deal of stigma attached to using sex toys and homemade vagina substitutes as masturbation aids, which is a total double standard as no one seems to bat an eyelid at the number of women who make out with Rabbit vibrators and condom-covered courgettes these days. Fortunately, the stigma doesn't stop all men doing it, but it can cause them to feel a little desperate or dirty, which taints what should be a wholeheartedly pleasurable experience.

I urge all the women on my plan to buy their men toys and actively encourage them to experiment. I even buy platonic male friends sex toys for Christmas and birthdays in an attempt to normalise their use (well, someone has to start the revolution), and I'm pleased to report they've gone down a treat.

4. How could they tell Pinocchio was lying?

Because his hand was on fire.

It's now time to separate the class. So, ladies, read on for Exercise B: Time to Reflect; gentlemen, head to page 23 for Exercise C: Great Explorations…

Exercise B

Time to Reflect (Women Only) – A Hands-on Solo Sex Lesson For Her

For the purposes of this exercise, I'd like you to be able to see your reflection – not only because it can help you identify the hot spots of your body that you can't normally see, but also because seeing yourself aroused provides an additional turn-on during masturbation. This helps you to grow fond of your figure, banishing insecurities over getting naked in front of others.

Any mirror you can sit comfortably in front of will do. If you can't find a mirror to admire yourself in, try this trick: position yourself on a chair or sofa in front of a TV screen. When a TV is switched off in a lit room the screen becomes reflective, but the finer details of your anatomy will be less clear, so use a small make-up compact or hand-held mirror for close-ups.

If you've ever read a sex manual before, you'll already know that you're meant to spend some time having a good, long look at your genitals in a mirror, thoroughly exploring your intimate components. You may think you're past all that, but it really is quite fascinating. Even if you've done this before, your body changes over time, so it's an ongoing education. It's also a brilliant way to monitor your health down there, as regular inspections will tell you whether any uncommon changes have taken place.

Getting to Know You

Massaging lubricant over your genitals before exploration will help your fingertips to glide more comfortably around the delicate skin there. If you don't have lubricant, use your own saliva as I take you on a guided tour . . .

Extra-curricular Activity
Lube patch test

When using a new lubricant for the first time (particularly if it's one that contains heating or cooling agents), do a skin patch test first. Dab a little of your chosen lube to the inside of your wrist and wait for twenty minutes to see whether your skin has an adverse reaction.

The mons, labia and clitoris

The vulva is the term for the external genitalia that you can see, often incorrectly referred to as the vagina. It begins at the top with your pubic mound – mons veneris, which translates as 'mountain of Venus' – a fatty pad of flesh, which also features on the male anatomy, and protects your pubic bones from crashing into each other during sex. Cleverly, the mons is also ergonomically designed to remain fleshed out regardless of weight, so even size zero celebs can have sex comfortably.

Now, banish all images of skinny celebrities thrashing around and stroke your fingertips across the contours of your genitals, parting your outer vaginal lips (labia majora) to fully reveal your inner lips (labia minora). The inner lips meet just below and above the clitoris. The clitoris, in blueprint, is much like the penis, only smaller. Notice how the clitoris has a hood; this is the female equivalent of a foreskin formed from the top of the inner lips. And just as the penis has a shaft, so does the clitoris. The head of the clitoris (glans clitoris) is the part you can see when the hood is retracted; the shaft, which is 2–4cm long, continues up from the head, just beneath the skin, towards the hair-covered pubic mound. It's attached to the pubic bone, but you can pinch it between your fingers and feel it move slightly. It then forks down into two roots (crura), which are 5–9cm long and run beneath the labia and also attach to the pubic bone. These roots may be sensitive to stimulation through the walls of the vagina and anus, and through the vulva. Scientists who don't believe in G-spots say that women who claim to have orgasms as a result of one may simply be having their internal clitorises stimulated.

The perineum, vestibule and urethra

In general terms, a vestibule is a hallway between an outer door and the main building; in genital terms it's the arched cavity you see when parting your inner lips and it houses the openings to your urethra and vagina. The urethral opening is sensitive in some women – stroke yours to see how it responds.

The perineum is the patch of skin between the vagina and anus, and some women find stimulating this spot incredibly arousing. Massage it to see how it feels for you.

Extra-curricular Activity

Boost your genital esteem

Several women suffer with what I call low genital esteem – unhappiness with the appearance or scent of their intimate parts. If you feel that way, it might help to artistically photograph, draw or paint a picture of your genitals to gain an appreciation of their unique feminine appeal.

It's also worth noting that several of the men I've interviewed for this book talk about enjoying the scent of a woman – not the sanitised, showered version, but the real heady smell of female genitalia. Inhale deeply while masturbating to pick up on this pheromone-packed thrill, and experience some of what he loves about your body.

The vagina and the G-spot

The vagina is the internal canal that leads to the cervix, rather than a collective term for the female genitalia. Inside your vagina, around five centimetres up on the front wall (the one nearest your stomach), you may be able to feel a raised, rippled nub of flesh, similar to a peach stone. This is your G-spot. Stroking it can bring on a sensation similar to wanting to pee, but by visiting the toilet prior to playtime, you can be confident you won't have any accidents.

Some women report that if they ride through this feeling, stimulating the G-spot can lead to female ejaculation – anything from a teaspoon to a teacup of clear fluid being ejaculated via the urethra. Though it may contain traces of urine – travelling, as it does, via the same passageway – it's not urine. Some doctors believe the fluid is produced in the Skene's gland, which is similar to the male prostate (the gland that produces semen). But don't get too caught up in the science – all that really matters here is what feels good for you. Being able to ejaculate doesn't necessarily increase the impact of orgasm, and the majority of women can't or don't do it, and are no worse off for it.

Another area to tease is the vaginal opening (introitus) as this area has one of the highest concentrations of nerve endings in the vagina. Try circling a finger around the entrance and then inserting several fingers at once to gently stretch it. All the while, keep looking at your reflection. As you become aroused you'll see changes in size, texture and colour as blood engorges your genitals and natural lubrication secretes through the vaginal walls. Also, the more turned on you get, the sexier you will look – that's because sexiness isn't about pouting and posing, it's about displaying raw desire, and that's something everyone can do, regardless of dress size.

Map Your Own Hot Spots

Now, it's playtime. Put down the mirror and get comfortable. You've identified the different components of your genitals, and as you go through the following selection of techniques, I'd like you to make a mental note of which areas are most sensitive and which strokes feel best for you. Breathe, relax and begin . . .

- **Tapping.** This brings blood to the skin's surface, enhancing sensation. So, firmly drum your fingers around your vaginal opening and then directly on the clitoral head where there is the greatest concentration of nerve endings. Note how this feels as the blood comes to the skin's surface. You can simultaneously clench and release your pelvic-floor muscles to enhance the feeling.

- **Wiping.** Sweep your whole hand, with fingers held rigid, from side to side across the vulva in a motion similar to an upside down windscreen wiper. This covers nerve endings in all the major hot spots: the clitoris, the vaginal opening and the labia. Experiment with different pressures and speeds to see what works best for you.

Extra-curricular Activity
Switch positions

Next time you masturbate, rather than opting for the most comfortable position, experiment with different stances: try masturbating standing up, kneeling on all fours, lying face-down or on your side. Varying positions will change the way your body responds to different techniques and you'll be aroused by the variety.

- **Plunging.** Some women prefer an up-and-down stroke, plunging their fingers down over the clitoris and urethra, then dipping them inside the vagina, before pulling the fingers back up again. This has the added bonus of transferring lots of the body's natural lubricant over the vulva with each stroke.

- **Circling.** Move your fingertips in circles around your vaginal entrance and then your clitoris, or you can join up the strokes to form a figure of eight around the vagina and clitoris. This suits women with more sensitive clitorises, as direct contact isn't made with the clitoral head. Try fantasising about your partner's tongue moving in the motion of your fingers as you go.

- **Pulling.** Pinching the labia together between outstretched fingers and then pulling them around and over the clitoris is another technique that works well for sensitive clitorises, with the soft padding of the labia cushioning each stroke.

This list of techniques is by no means exhaustive; I fully expect you

Course Notes
Wander lust

While experimenting with solo sex techniques, allow your free hand to wander. Twirl a nipple, pull on your pubic hair, grip your inner thighs or massage your abdomen – whatever feels good. Busy hands are always better placed to find hidden orgasm triggers.

to discover some new moves yourself as you explore my self-pleasuring suggestions. Just be sure to make a mental note of any new tricks you enjoy, not only for your next solo sex session, but also for when you're with your partner – you now have a lot to teach him.

Penetration for One

We'll play with sex aids in more depth on Day Five, but for now, I'd like to discuss their role in solo sexploration. You may already own a Rabbit-style vibrator, or something similar featuring a shaft with a vibrating unit attached, but I suggest using a separate dildo and vibrating bullet in this exercise, so you can isolate and appreciate the sensations of each.

If you don't own a vibrating bullet (or similar), use the tip of a standard vibrator, or even an electric toothbrush with the head removed and a flannel around the tip. If you don't have a dildo, vegetables such as carrots or courgettes make great substitutes. You can even buy a selection in different sizes to discover exactly which sizes work best for you, before finally investing in a dildo that will be a perfect fit. Wash the veg and cover it with a condom to protect yourself from the transfer of pesticides and bacteria, then coat your homemade playmate in lube before sliding it inside your vagina. Courgettes tend to have a natural curve so you can point the tip towards the front wall of your vagina to stimulate your G-spot; this should prove easier than trying to reach this awkwardly placed hot spot with your fingers.

First, lubricate your dildo and slowly slide it inside you; note the sensation of the vaginal entrance stretching. Around another five

Real Sex
Cucumber Dip

My favourite homemade sex aid is a cucumber dildo. Cucumbers are girthy and I'm a bit of a size queen; they're also a bit more malleable than carrots, so they feel more real, and once peeled they're naturally wet and juicy so you don't need any more lube. If you use them straight from the fridge, the cool sensation is strange, but quite pleasant. If you're going for real feel, don't refrigerate them first.

Amanda, 32

centimetres inside the vagina, your dildo will pass your G-spot on the front wall of the vagina. Point the tip of your toy at this erogenous zone and massage it, using firm strokes, either circling the G-spot or rubbing up and down over the top of it. The G-spot will swell as it's stimulated, making it easier to locate.

When sampling your body's responses, be aware that the more aroused you are, the more sensation you'll feel. If something doesn't feel amazing at first, try it again when you're more turned on. If you're having trouble feeling aroused, take some time to fantasise and stroke your most responsive erogenous zone (usually the clitoris) before returning to uncharted territories.

Extra-curricular Activity
Sweet talk

It is not uncommon to concentrate unconsciously on being quiet during masturbation. This may be because, for many of us, our first solo sex experiences occurred when we were young and still living in our parents' homes where we needed to be quiet to avoid getting 'caught'. This becomes habit-forming, so that we lose the ability to be vocal at all during sex. Now is a good time to start breaking that habit during masturbation. Start by telling yourself what feels good; bring in a few X-rated terms and see how liberating that feels.

Next, we're heading for the 'A-spot', or anterior fornix, located at the top of the front wall of the vagina close to the cervix. Massaging this spot will increase lubrication. Then on to the cervix or 'C-spot' (the opening of the womb), which is sensitive in some women who enjoy rhythmically prodding or stroking it. Depending on your size, you may need quite a long dildo to put this to the test, but be warned that many women find the experience uncomfortable. If you discover you feel the same, don't be disappointed. It means the exercise has been a success in uncovering exactly what does *and* doesn't work for you.

Now you've located the commonly known internal erogenous zones, see if you can find others that are unique to you. Also, think about the techniques you enjoy. Do you like to clench and grip your toy with your pelvic muscles? Do you prefer to slowly slide it in and out? Or do short fast thrusts turn you on?

Once you've revelled in the delights of your dildo, put it to one side and introduce your vibrating bullet. Don't take it straight to your clitoris; tease your body first. Start rolling the bullet over your nipples. One per cent of the female population can climax through nipple play alone; the majority aren't that lucky, but the sensation can still send shock waves of sexual tension straight to your genitals.

Next, roll it down over your abdomen, remembering to keep your breathing steady and deep, then take the bullet around your labia and down to your perineum. Vibrations here can travel to the deep roots of your clitoris, and also stimulate the anal nerves, which are highly responsive (but make sure you don't place the bullet in or over your anus, as you can transfer bacteria from here back to your vagina).

When you bring the bullet back up to your vagina, dip it inside you. Focus on the sensation, and maintain your breathing. Finally, run the vibe up to your clitoris. Having fun yet?

Now I'd like you to reintroduce your dildo, while continuing to play with your vibe. You can simply leave your toy inside of you for a feeling of fullness, clench and release it with your pelvic muscles or slowly slide it in and out. At the same time, focus vibrations on your clitoris. Clitorises adore vibrations, but everyone is different: some women like to retract the hood for the most intense level of sensation; others like vibrations just to the left or right of it; and some prefer to close their legs and have the vibrations run through their labia.

I didn't save the clitoral stimulation until last because it's the best; I did it because statistically, it's the type of stimulation that is most likely to trigger orgasm and, when you consider that an orgasm only lasts ten seconds or so, it seems illogical to make it the entire focus of sex. The building of sexual tension – which takes up the most part – should be savoured too. Once you appreciate that, you've successfully completed the exercise.

For those who want to explore further, there's another element of solo sex that we haven't yet discussed involving anal play – see Exercise D: Bottom of the Class, p. 28, if you're feeling adventurous . . .

Exercise C

Great Explorations (Men Only) – A Hands-on Solo Sex Lesson For Him

You may be wondering what a woman can possibly teach a man about male masturbation? Well, quite a lot actually. Despite the fact that the majority of men have had healthy, long-term relationships with their manhood, heterosexual males only know about their *own* penises, and – as with any long-term relationship – it's easy to become stuck in a rut. So for you, Day One of my plan is about changing your usual routine. If one of the following styles is your own, please don't use it for this exercise. The goal is to discover new techniques, become less reliant on one tried-and-tested method (and therefore more responsive to partner sex) and to increase the wow factor of your orgasms. But first you need the magic ingredient . . .

Let's Get Wet

A male porn star once told me that if you've masturbated with lubricant, you'll never look back. I've found his theory to be true time and time again. The warmth and wetness of lubricant enhances sensation and provides a more 'real-feel' experience to boost fantasies.

It's also a fact that some of the more intricate male masturbation techniques are either impossible or incredibly painful without lubricant. So, make sure you have some to hand before experimenting with new strokes. There are lots of lubricants to choose from on today's market. Take your pick:

- **Cooling lube** – usually enhanced with menthol, the formula causes the skin to tingle; a perfect choice for any man who also likes the sensation of playing with ice. Alternatively, coat your penis in a standard, water-based lube, and hold an ice cube in the palm of your hand. As the ice melts you'll have the added bonus of the water replenishing the lubricant, so that there's no need to reapply.

- **Warming lube** – designed to heat up delicate flesh, these lubes use active ingredients like cinnamon bark. The effect can be too intense for some penises, and it's always advisable to do a skin patch test on your wrist first. If you begin to feel uncomfortable after applying, wash the area in cold water immediately. If you have sensitive skin, use a standard, water-based lube that you've warmed by floating the tube in a bowl of hot water or by placing it on a radiator – but *always* check that the temperature is acceptable by dabbing some on the thin skin of your wrist before pouring it on your manhood.

> ### Course Notes
> # Clear choice
>
> When selecting a new lubricant, opt for a clear non-staining variety, otherwise your sheets will tell the story. If you're new to lube, rather than investing in one bottle, buy a sample pack – many reputable brands sell them. If you don't have any lube, try a good-quality organic body or food oil (olive oil is good to the skin, and a lot of men swear by Vaseline), but only if you don't intend to have sex before your next shower: anything other than good-quality, purpose-made water-based or silicone-based lubricant will upset the delicate pH balance of a vagina and oil may cause a latex condom to tear.

- **Flavoured lube** – available in flavours as diverse as 'pina colada' and 'chocolate cherry', these lubes are a little wasted on solo sex sessions, but are handy all-rounders as they're condom-compatible and an interesting condiment for oral sex.

- **Standard, water-based lube** – the most commonly sold lubricant, as it's the most versatile (cooling, heating and flavoured lubes are usually all water-based), and it can be used with condoms. Complaints against water-based lube include a feeling of stickiness after a while and that it can dry up too quickly, although a drop of water replenishes it, so keep a glass to hand.

- **Silicone-based lube** – this is long lasting, and doesn't wash off with water alone, making it great for solo sex in the bath or shower. It's also a lot of people's choice for anal play because of its durability and condom-compatibility. It's usually more expensive than water-based lubricants, but that's precisely because a little goes a long way. However, it can't be used with silicone masturbation aids as it erodes silicone material.

- **Oil-based lube** – again, lasts longer than water-based lube and there are a lot of brands on the market designed purely for male masturbation; not safe to use with latex condoms, however, as oil erodes latex.

Real Sex
Secret Voyeur

When my husband thinks I'm asleep, he'll play with himself in bed. I'm not embarrassed to confront him about it – we have a very honest, open relationship – but I enjoy the feeling of him moving beside me, and the tension in my body as I try to lie still as the undetected voyeur. Part of me wants to roll over and grab him, but part of me enjoys these 'secret' moments he has. Then, afterwards, when he's asleep, I do the same.

Elizabeth, 48

Playtime

Now you've selected your lube, it's time to try some new techniques. It's surprising how few men know the terms for the components that make up the head of the penis, so here's a quick guide:

- **Glans** – head of the penis
- **Urethra** – opening in the end of the penis
- **Corona** – ridge around the underside of the head of the penis
- **Frenulum** – the thin membranous skin that attaches the foreskin to the glans

Remember, the aim of the game is discovery, so avoid tried-and-tested methods and play with those you don't already know. When you practise these new techniques, also try watching yourself in front of a large mirror. Take in the way your arms move, the look in your eyes, the expression on your face and the tensing of your thighs. All of these are a major turn-on to women. See what they see, and enjoy your body.

Real Sex
Wake-up Call

Sometimes, when I'm too tired to have sex and my man's horny, he'll masturbate in front of me. Generally speaking, I only have to watch him for a few minutes before my tiredness passes and I want to join in. There's something intimate about watching him stroke himself, so even if I'm not in the mood, it's a pleasure to watch him do it.

Emma, 33

- **The corkscrew.** Once it is erect, steady your shaft by gripping it at the base, between the fingers of your left hand, then wrap your right palm around the upside of the shaft at the base (so the palm is facing away from you) and slide that hand to the tip of your penis, twisting it around the head until your palm faces up towards you. From here slide your palm down the underside of the shaft to the base, then grip the base with your fingers, while repeating the same move using your left hand. It takes a while to master, but after a few repetitions you'll pick up the pace and it's well worth it when you do – the sensation of your palm sweeping over the head of your penis will feel divine.

- **The continuous stroke.** Make a fist around the glans, then stroke down the shaft from tip to base with one hand, quickly followed by the other, making sure both hands are working the penis at all times. The aim is to create the sensation of one long continuous stroke or the feeling of plunging into a never-ending well of flesh.

- **The fire-starter.** Place your penis between your hands, then rub your hands together as though rubbing a piece of wood to start a fire. Work up and down the shaft in this way, and pay particular attention to the glans.

- **Polishing.** You'll need a lot of lube for this one to prevent you from over-stretching your frenulum. Hold your penis at the base and position it so it's flat on your stomach; with your other hand held flat and rigid, stroke your palm back and forth over your glans and frenulum.

Extra-curricular Activity

Ball games

As a prelude to masturbation, or even during it, try massaging your testicles: cover them in lube and roll each one between your fingertips; this is also a great way to check the area for any lumps and bumps and detect any changes as soon as they occur, so make a habit of it.

- **Tap 'n' tickle.** Again, hold your penis at the base and position it so it's flat on your stomach. Then take your other hand and quickly drum all your fingers across the frenulum and corona, almost as though you're tickling them. The tapping will bring blood to the surface of the skin, while the tickling will feel like little licks.

- **Pearl necklace.** Borrow some pearls or beads from your girlfriend or wife. Check there aren't any rough seams around the beads (better check they aren't a family heirloom first, too), then wrap them around your shaft and roll them up and down over your shaft and corona for textured self-pleasure.

Real Sex

Gay Parade

I watch a lot of gay porn because it's the only place that I get to see decent shots of men masturbating. There's something so hot about seeing a guy swell as he gets closer to orgasm, and the look on his face when he comes is amazing. My boyfriend thinks it's weird, but he watches women masturbate in porn films so I don't see how this is any different.

Leanne, 30

The above represents just a brief selection of techniques designed to work as foreplay to your usual method, prolonging the build-up to – and therefore the power of – your orgasm. Once you've experienced and appreciated a more scenic route to climax, you have successfully completed Day One of my plan.

For those who are still feeling adventurous, there's another element of solo sex that we haven't yet explored involving anal stimulation. A lot of straight men are getting in on the act these days, so if you're prepared to go further, read on . . .

Exercise D

Bottom of the Class (Optional) – A Guide to Anal Masturbation

Though few people talk about it, everyone has an opinion on anal sex. Some people swear it gives them the deepest full-body orgasms going, others think it's painful, unhygienic, 'dirty' (in the deviant sense), sinful, unnatural or something that only homosexual men can enjoy.

If a particular sex act makes you feel uncomfortable or turns you off, you shouldn't force yourself or *be* forced into doing it, which is why this exercise is optional. However, you should know that anal sex is only painful when it's done incorrectly, and it can be carried out safely and hygienically with condoms, lubricant and the correct techniques.

It also has to be noted that, regardless of sexual persuasion, all men are built the same way, with the same system of nerve endings, so there's no logical reason why heterosexual men should not enjoy the sensations that homosexual men do, not to mention the same freedom, in the sense that gay men decide whether they enjoy anal penetration based on preference rather than preconceptions.

Also note that for women, many of the anxieties about anal sex are similar to those they have about vaginal sex prior to losing their virginity, which do disappear once they've got the hang of it.

I suggest that if you wish to experience anal penetration, you should explore alone first. This prevents embarrassment and means that you're more able to relax. It also means you are completely in control, so there's less chance of causing yourself any pain.

Tools of the Tradesmen's Entrance

The right equipment is essential in anal play; using the wrong kit can end up in an embarrassing trip to the Accident and Emergency department, so please don't take that risk. You will need:

- **Lubricant.** Always use lubricant for any kind of anal play. If you're dressing your finger or toy in a condom, use a water-based or silicone-based lubricant (but don't apply silicone lube on to silicone toys). If you aren't using condoms you can experiment with good-quality, purpose-made, oil-based lubes, which some people prefer for anal play.

- **Clean hands.** Beginners most often use their own fingers. Hands should be thoroughly washed, nails should be trimmed, and, if you feel squeamish about entering this area of your body, you can pop a condom on your finger to prevent direct contact. Before entry, fingers should, of course, be lubricated.

- **Accessories.** Butt plugs (sold online and in adult stores) are the most popular style of toy specially designed for anal play (you will learn about the rest on Day Five). Unlike dildos, standard butt plugs have a flared base beneath an indented ridge that prevents them from being completely sucked up into the rectum when the anal muscles contract.

  If you don't have a butt plug, a 15cm carrot with a wide base can provide a homemade alternative. Peel and wash the carrot, carve a ridge around the circumference, about 4cm from the base, then cover the carrot with a condom, and voilà – a homemade butt plug. Lubricate and prepare to insert.

Note: women's health warning – *never* put anything inside the vagina that has been in your rear – the transfer of bacteria can cause infection.

Going Where the Sun Don't Shine

To relax your anus, cover its rim with lube and massage around the opening in small, firm, circular strokes – the nerve endings should tingle in response to your touch.

When you're ready to go further, slowly slide the tip of your finger or toy inside you. Your muscles will involuntarily contract – this is natural – and after a few moments they will relax again so you can slide further inside.

You should feel no pain. If you do, you may need more lubricant, or your body may be too tense. To relax, take deep breaths, think sexy thoughts, use your free hand to masturbate in your usual way for a while, and apply more lube just to be on the safe side. Once you're comfortable again, try going a little deeper, until you've fully inserted your finger or butt plug (up to the ridge).

The male G-spot

The prostate – also known as the male G-spot – is a small gland, about the size and shape of a quail's egg. The testicles produce sperm, which is carried to the prostate where it mixes with seminal fluid. The resulting concoction is what a man ejaculates when he orgasms.

Some men enjoy the sensation of having pressure applied to the prostate. To try it, a man should insert his index finger into his anus up to around his second knuckle – until he feels the prostate through the front rectal wall – then press towards his pelvis in a firm 'come-hither' motion.

Some men like to massage their prostate; both men and women may enjoy the sensation of a toy or finger slowing thrusting in and out of the anus, while others simply enjoy the feeling of fullness in their rectum, while continuing to masturbate in the usual way – generally speaking, anal play works best in conjunction with another form of stimulation. Once you've found your favourite combo, masturbate to orgasm. Afterwards, you can make an informed decision on whether or not you want to make it a part of your sexual repertoire.

Congratulations on completing Day One of *7 Days to Amazing Sex*. You've mastered the art of masturbation and learnt how to use your hands as sexual playthings. Now you're ready to let those hands loose on your partner.

Day Two
Strokes of Genius

On Day One of *7 Days to Amazing Sex*, you learnt how to pleasure yourself by hand. Now you're going to learn how to use your hands to pleasure your partner.

As you'll be working together, I have to stress that, no matter how tempted you are, or how turned on you become, it's important to limit your activities to hand play only.

Full penetrative sex is strictly forbidden until Day Four. This allows for a build-up of sexual tension, the development of new sexual skills and a clear break from the habitual routine of your old sex life. Too often, penetrative sex is seen as the 'main course' of any sexual encounter. This baffles me as there are so many sexual options on the menu, and yet large numbers of the sexual complaints I hear are from people who are bored by a lack variety in their sex lives.

You can instantly add an element of surprise and novelty to sex by simply breaking away from your old routine – which for many couples involves a set allocation of minutes for foreplay followed by penetrative sex and then sleep. Sound familiar?

The key is to make all the sex acts on the menu work for you. And listen to your body: some days you might feel more inclined towards oral sex, while on others you may prefer manual stimulation, and there may be days when penetrative sex is what you crave. And, of course, you can combine all of the above in whatever format you fancy.

Our hands are the most versatile sexual tools we have. They can grip at whatever pressure is preferred, they can penetrate and stroke and they can reach parts of the body that aren't always stimulated during oral or penetrative sex. And I'm going to show you how to use these tools like a pro.

Real Sex
Give the Girl a Hand

While I really enjoy oral sex and standard sex in just about every position, when it comes to reaching a climax I need fingers. For me, fingers are capable of so much more than tongues or penises as they're so versatile; they can be hard or soft, and they can reach all my nooks and crannies. I like to lie back and feel all four of my partner's fingers rubbing across my clitoris while he uses his other hand to penetrate me, or tug on my nipples at the same time – that always makes me come. If we're in a rear-entry position, he can reach around with his hand to stroke my clitoris instead, but when he's using only his hands, all his focus is on me and that's what really rocks my world.

Mae, 30

Exercise A
Meet the Genitals – How Well Do You Know Each Other's 'Private Parts'?

You may think you know your partner's genitals like the back of your hand. You've no doubt seen them often enough, and felt them often enough to have a general idea about what's down there. But have you ever really got up close and personal with them, other than when you're in the heat of the moment, a time when your powers of concentration are most likely compromised? Have you ever had a guided tour? Do you even know what your partner calls the different components of their 'private parts'?

The following exercise will help you to identify the specific erogenous zones of your partner's genitals and use terminology that you're both comfortable with to describe them. This will enable you to communicate your desires clearly and specifically, guaranteeing better sex.

Step 1: Have You Guessed What It Is Yet?

Have you guessed what it is yet? First, let's test your anatomical knowledge of the opposite sex. Over the page, you'll find two diagrams: one showing female genitalia, the other, male genitalia. Without peeking at the answers at the end of the exercise, fill in the anatomical names of each of the genital components in the spaces provided (men should fill in the Female Genitals diagram, while women should fill in the Male Genitals diagram). Feel free to help each other out. The areas you're aiming to identify are:

- **On her** – inner labia, clitoris, mons veneris, vagina, outer labia, urethra.
- **On him** – shaft, median raphe, mons pubis, glans, urethra, frenulum, testicles, corona, foreskin, scrotum.

It doesn't matter if you don't get them all right. Think of it as a meet 'n' greet exercise. What's important is that you become aware of the different buttons to push between your partner's legs. While the clitoris on women and the glans on men tend to be the most sensitive spots, there may be other hot spots that crave attention, or the obvious ones may be so sensitive that your lover prefers to be touched next to, rather than directly on them. Ultimately, the better acquainted you are with your lover's genitals, the better you will be as a lover, so get your pens out and start plotting.

Female Genitals

A. _____

B. _____

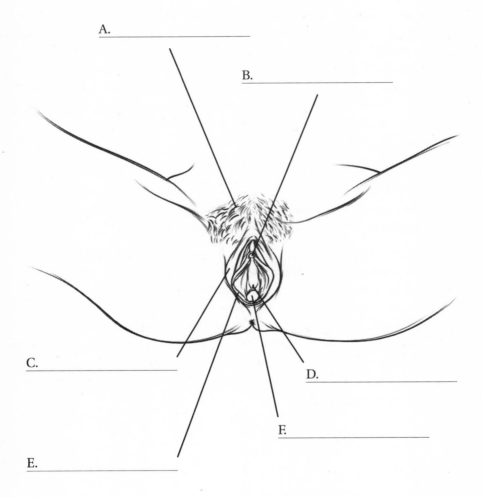

C. _____

D. _____

F. _____

E. _____

Male Genitals

A. _____

B. _____

C. _____

D. _____

F. _____

E. _____

G. _____

H. _____

J. _____

I. _____

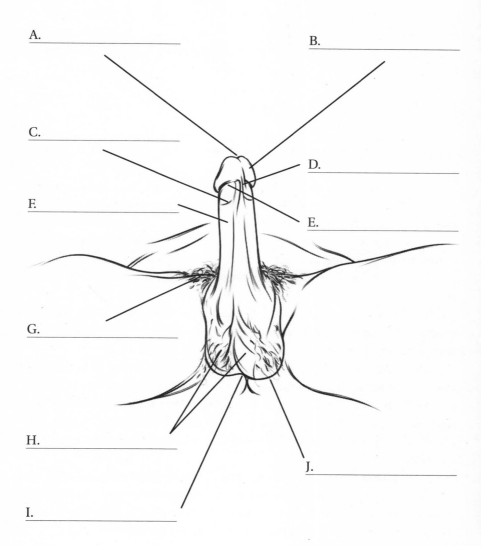

Answers

Female Genitals

A. Mons veneris
B. Clitoris
C. Outer labia
D. Urethra
E. Inner labia
F. Vagina

Male Genitals

A. Urethra
B. Glans
C. Foreskin (retracted)
D. Frenulum
E. Corona
F. Shaft

G. Mons pubis
H. Testicles
I. Median raphe
J. Scrotum

Step 2: The Name Game

Now you're up to speed on the anatomical terminology, you can say, 'Honey, I like it when you flick your tongue over my urethra,' or 'I'm most sensitive where my frenulum meets my corona,' and you'll both know exactly what you're talking about. But the trouble with anatomical terms is that they can sound cold and clinical – that's fine when you're having a candid conversation out of the bedroom, but during sex it can be a turn-off.

The alternative is to use slang or pet terms, but what's a sexy word to one person may be a total passion-killer to another, and that's where this lesson comes in.

Ladies, go back to the Female Genitals diagram and next to your partner's answers write the name you want him to use to describe that part of your body. You can write more than one option if you wish, but make sure it sounds sexy to you. For example, for the word clitoris, you may find it sexier to use the abbreviation 'clit', or a euphemism such as 'button'.

Gents, please follow suit, filling in the Male Genitals diagram with the terms you would like your partner to use. When you're both done, make a mental note of these terms. Think of them as your sex dictionary and use them not only to guide, but also to arouse each other.

Step 3: 'X' Marks the Spot

For the final part of this exercise, I'd like you both to mark on your diagrams the areas you like to have stimulated. Use a little cross to pinpoint your hot spots. Having identified these areas on Day One of my plan when you were working alone, you can now share this information with your partner.

Couples often find it easier to discuss their genitals in this way, rather than when they're naked using their own nether regions for reference; it feels safer as there's less risk of embarrassment and this will help you both to be more open. Don't hold back – this is your chance to get exactly what you want in bed.

Also, you're not restricted to marking areas already listed on the diagrams. For example, a woman may feel deliciously sensitive just to the left of her clitoris, while a man might like a tight grip around the very base of his penis. Wherever you want to be touched, let 'X' mark the spot – and remember you can both refer back to these diagrams at any time.

Armed with new-found information about your lover's erogenous zones, it's now time to move on to the next exercise, for which you'll need lots of lubricant.

Extra-curricular Activity
Play on words

If you've never talked openly in much detail about your genitals, you probably haven't given arousing terminology much thought either. If that's the case, spare some time now to write a list of all the names you find appropriate. Discuss with your partner those terms you'd like to use in the bedroom, starting with terms for penis and vulva (the collective term for the external female genitalia). How about Tantric terms such as 'lingham' and 'yoni'? Or metaphors such as 'sword' and 'flower'? You can then go on to name the more intimate components. For example, if you both like the term 'flower' for vulva, how about 'petals' for labia and 'bud' for clitoris? Once you've developed your own secret sex language, you'll be fluent in the bedroom.

Exercise B

Arousal Massage – The Art of Arousal Without Genital Contact

I would suggest men carry out the following exercise first. This is because women are less likely to feel tired after orgasm (and orgasm *is* the likely outcome of these exercises, though it's not the ultimate goal). However, if you'd prefer to flip the order, then feel free to do so. Once you've decided who will go first, you can proceed.

In this exercise you'll continue working together, taking turns to use nothing but your hands to pleasure each other. As I've already explained, manual stimulation doesn't have to be confined to 'foreplay', and can be the main event in any hot sex session – but the act itself *does* require foreplay. Don't instantly reach for hot spots your partner pointed out to you in the previous exercise; you need first to tease open their mind, then their body, to the possibility of arousal, and one of the best ways to do this is through arousal massage.

Allow at least fifteen minutes for arousal massage. To begin, your partner should be lying face-down on a comfortable surface such as a bed, feeling totally at ease. Here's a list of things to check:

- Can you see a clock? Amateur masseuses often underestimate the time they've spent on massage and it's essential that this process isn't rushed.

- Is the room warm enough?

- Is the lighting soft and ambient?

- Have you eliminated potential distractions – switched off mobile phones and set the landline phone ringer to silent, for example?

- Does your partner need the bathroom? Toilet visits are always advisable prior to intimacy.

- Does your partner like music playing in the background?

- Are your hands warm?

- Is your partner lying comfortably?

- Are you able to reach all their contours and the massage lotion?

Once the scene is set and your partner is comfortable, you're ready to begin.

Bottom Strokes

Apply lots of lubricant to your hands, then rub them together to warm the lotion. You can use a two-in-one massage lotion-cum-lubricant for this exercise, or you can use any standard massage lotion, but wash your hands and switch to water-based lube for the genitals (fragranced oils and lotions can have an adverse reaction on our intimate bits).

Now, place your hands firmly against your partner's buttocks with your fingers pointing up towards their shoulders. From here, move the heels of your hands in very firm outward circular motions, up and over the cheeks of their bottom, parting them with each stroke. After fifteen to thirty slow strokes, switch from the heels of your hands to your thumbs for a more intense sensation.

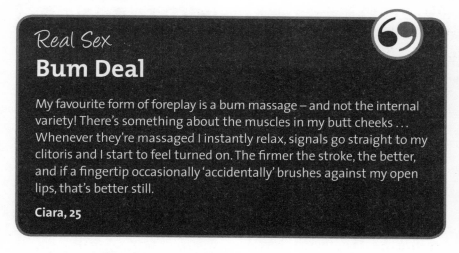

Real Sex
Bum Deal

My favourite form of foreplay is a bum massage – and not the internal variety! There's something about the muscles in my butt cheeks . . . Whenever they're massaged I instantly relax, signals go straight to my clitoris and I start to feel turned on. The firmer the stroke, the better, and if a fingertip occasionally 'accidentally' brushes against my open lips, that's better still.

Ciara, 25

In women, these motions cause the labia to open and close, gently and repeatedly 'kissing' the clitoris within, awakening its senses and making it want more. In men, the strokes will reverberate through the gluteus muscles to their prostate (the male G-spot) embedded within the rectal wall, arousing the sensitive nerves there.

The key is to work very, *very* slowly, being careful to never actually touch the genitals, but always tease them with the presence of your hands.

Ask how the pressure feels. Would they like more or less, or is it just right?

To heighten sensitivity in the skin, vary your technique occasionally by following firm strokes with the light tracing of your fingertips.

Hamstring Strokes

Work up to the small of your partner's back, circling your thumbs out from the either side of the spine, then work back down over the bottom and down to the back of the knees, never losing contact with their body for any reason other than to apply more massage lotion or lubricant. When you reach the back of their knees, gently part their legs – your left hand should be working their left leg, your right hand should be on their right leg.

Using the same outward circles, mixed with occasional light fingertip traces, massage all the way back up the hamstring muscles, taking your time to finally reach around to the inner thighs – erogenous zones in their own right. Don't be tempted to go any further – genital contact will feel far more delicious when your partner has been made to wait for it.

Flip, then Knees to Hips

Now, quietly ask your partner to turn over so they're lying on their back. Using the same simple strokes, begin the massage at just above the knees, working up to the hips. This is another popular hot spot on the human anatomy, but due to the high concentration of nerve endings, they may also find this a ticklish area, so keep pressure firm.

Course Notes
The unpredictability factor

One of the major delights of being masturbated by someone else is the fact that it's unpredictable, so that your skin's senses are heightened as they try to anticipate the next move. Over the following pages, you'll both learn and develop some signature hand techniques to push your each other's buttons, which is great news for your sex life. However, if from this day on you only ever follow the tried-and-tested format of the signature moves you learn today, as much as they feel great for your partner now, you'll lose your exciting 'unpredictability factor'. Remember, in the build-up to orgasm, there's always room to experiment with new moves.

Abs to Mons

Next, move your hands to the lower abdomen. The area between the navel and genitals is revered as a major erogenous zone in many cultures, but so many people completely overlook it. Slowly sweep the palms of your hands from the centre of the abdomen out to the hips for ten to twenty strokes, then circle your thumbs over the mons veneris (in women) or mons pubis (in the men) – the fleshy mound covering the pubic bone.

By now, your partner's body should be relaxed and aroused, and you're ready to move on to the next exercise.

Exercise C

Pleasuring Her By Hand (Men Only) – A Guide to Manually Pleasing Women

Throughout this exercise you need to ensure your hands remain sufficiently lubricated, without being so wet that the sensation of friction is lost. It's easy to upset the delicate pH balance of the female genitals with fragranced body oils, so if you were using one, wash your hands and switch to a water-based lube now. When it starts to dry out you can replenish it with a few drops of water, or simply apply a little more. You can also dip your fingers inside her vagina to spread her natural lubrication over her clitoris and the rest of her vulva.

A word about your nails: they should be trimmed so that no more than 1mm of white nail tip is showing, and smooth and as

Course Notes

Ego massage

As well as massaging her labia, you may also need to massage her ego! Not all women will feel comfortable lying open-legged with their genitalia in full view, so reassure your partner that her intimate areas look, smell and feel beautiful to you. You could even dip a finger inside of her and then suck it to show just how much you want her.

pristinely clean as a surgeon's – your hands will be entering her body after all, plus grubby hands are a total turn-off.

Like men, most women appreciate a repetitive stroke as they approach climax, so build arousal and sexual tension with a variety of techniques, then adopt the most pleasurable stroke for her and rhythmically build momentum to a consistent speed and pressure that takes her to orgasm. Some women will climax from a slow and gentle touch, while others will prefer firmer, faster strokes. No two women are the same, so don't assume that what worked for a previous lover will also work for your current partner. Instead, monitor her responses through the following:

1. **Sexual body language.** Being able to read her sexual body language is a valuable (and easily learnt) skill. Visible signs of arousal include the swelling of breasts, the swelling and reddening of the labia, a sex rash (flushing of skin often seen around the décolletage) and increased lubrication – though when you're using lubricant this can be difficult to detect. More obvious signs may include rapid breathing, moaning and the movement of her hips. For example, if she's thrusting her hips and genitals towards your hand, she's probably ready for more pressure, and if she's pulling away, she probably wants less.

2. **Verbal communication.** Even couples who prefer to not mix sex and conversation should be vocal occasionally. It isn't necessary to have a running commentary, and for some that would be a complete turn-off, but non-verbal communication isn't always enough to clearly understand what your partner wants, particularly when you're still only just learning to read their sexual body language. To encourage a reticent lover to speak up, keep your voice low and soft and whisper questions like, 'Does that feel good?', 'Would you like me to slow down?' and, 'Do you want it harder?'

Continuing from the arousal massage where you were circling your thumbs over her mons, I'd now like you to move into genital massage by slowly stroking your thumbs down either side of her labia to beneath her vaginal opening, then back up again. Repeat this move ten to fifteen times before finally moving between the labia. This gives you time to really look at her genitals and the positioning of their components, which you identified on the diagram earlier today. At the same time, it feels wonderfully soothing and arousing for her.

Basic Clitoral Strokes

On Day One, women were asked to experiment with different basic masturbation techniques for the clitoris including moving fingers across it from side to side, plunging fingers up and down over it and circling fingertips around it. Ask your partner which techniques she most enjoyed, then try them yourself.

If you're having difficulty getting the pressure and pace right, ask your partner to place her hand over the top of yours so she can guide you until you've found your rhythm. You may need to alter your position to get it right. Conversely, as you're able to approach her genitals from a different vantage point, the impact of each technique could vary in a good way and she could find you're able to pleasure her in ways she could never do herself.

Finally, think about how you masturbate yourself. In blueprint, the head of the clitoris is similar to the head of the penis and a similar rhythm may feel divine.

Penetration and the G-spot

While the clitoris is proven to have the highest concentration of nerve endings anywhere in the genitalia (and, indeed, the human body), there are other pleasure spots to explore. The entrance to the vagina is particularly sensitive in some women; try circling the outer opening with your fingertips before sliding inside.

Around five centimetres up, embedded in the front wall of the vaginal canal (stomach-side) you'll come across the G-spot, a nub of rippled flesh that feels like a soft peach stone. The more turned on she is, the more swollen and

Course Notes
Ejaculation theory

All too often, when men learn about female ejaculation, they instantly want to create that response in their partners. They become goal-orientated, in the belief that causing ejaculation makes them better lovers. It doesn't. The majority of women don't ejaculate, and they're no less orgasmic for it. If you become too focused on trying to achieve this end, the partner who simply cannot ejaculate may start to feel like she's a disappointment to you sexually, and, rather than turning her on, you'll quickly turn her off.

therefore apparent it will be, so seek it out after she's shown clear signs of arousal.

It can be awkward for a woman to reach her own G-spot without using tailor-made toys, but for you it will be much easier. To stimulate this spot, with your palm facing upwards, slightly hook your fingers and move them back and forth over her G-spot in a firm 'come-hither' motion. Ask her how that feels.

Not all women enjoy G-spot stimulation so don't be offended or disheartened if she has no reaction to this technique. Some women may experience a sensation like they need to pee because the G-spot is close to their bladder. This can obviously be off-putting for her, but, assuming she's emptied her bladder before this exercise, it's highly unlikely that there'll be any accidents.

Real Sex

G-orgasms

I'd always found it relatively easy to climax during sex, but I didn't have a G-spot orgasm until I was in my late twenties. The guy I was dating was really into female ejaculation and spent ages pressing into my G-spot hard with his fingers until I squirted. I felt a kind of muscular pulsing deep in my vagina too, which was nice enough, but nothing compared to a clitoral orgasm. Annoyingly, since then, I tend to ejaculate every time I have sex – though that could be because my man is well endowed. It's as if the ejaculation part of me was unblocked by that other guy, and now I can't stop it, which is a nightmare on the sheets! If you ask me, G-spot orgasms are overrated. They can be nice when you have a clitoral orgasm at the same time, but they're better as an enhancement to a 'normal' orgasm than as an orgasm in their own right.

Jenny, 34

If your partner can override that feeling, she may go on to experience deeper sensations; some women say G-spot stimulation gives them 'full-body orgasms' – orgasmic sensations all over their body rather than the localised sensation of climax felt in the genitals. Others experience female ejaculation – up to half a teacup of clear fluid expelled from the body via the urethra. For the majority of women, however, simply the feeling of fullness in their vagina, or that 'full' feeling combined with a thrusting stroke, is orgasmic enough. Insert as many well-lubricated fingers as she's comfortable with.

While penetrating her with your fingers in this position, you can also place your thumb over her clitoris – stroke your thumb from side to side or up and down over it while you stimulate her internally for double the thrills.

Multi-tasking

When it comes to your hands, one of their major assets in sexual terms is the fact that there are two of them – they're a veritable one-man ménage à trois! When one hand is working her clitoris, your other hand should never be idle. You can use it to pleasure her vaginally, play with her breasts or penetrate her rear with a very well-lubricated finger (but make sure you give her some warning first).

However, if you've tried to rub your stomach and pat your head at the same time, you'll know that it's difficult to get your hands to act in opposing ways. Instead, try to work with your hands' symmetry. For example, if you're thrusting the fingers of your left hand inside your partner, follow the up-and-down motion with the thumb of your right hand rubbing over her clitoris in the same direction.

Real Sex
The Handshake

I was having sex with my girlfriend doggy-style, but I knew I couldn't last much longer and she was nowhere near coming, so I pulled out and used my fingers instead; I put my first two fingers inside her, then twisted my hand from left to right, which meant I was stroking her bum with my thumb while my last two fingers swished against her clitoris. She came really quickly and said it was the best hand-job she'd ever had. I do it all the time now.

Nathan, 23

Hand-play Positions

For the duration of this exercise your partner has been laying on her back, this being commonly accepted as the most comfortable masturbation position. However, angling her body in different ways will allow for different sensations. Experiment with positions – she could try lying on her side, standing or kneeling on all fours. Once in a new position, try different hand-play techniques. For example, standing behind her you could put one hand between her legs and penetrate from behind, bringing your other hand around her body to stroke her clitoris at the same time.

When you've experimented with new positions and techniques, treat your lover to her favourite combo to take her all the way to climax. But remember: it's hand play only today and you're not permitted to indulge in any other acts at this stage. Also, don't feel disappointed if your partner doesn't climax – if you've experimented thoroughly, you will have changed tempo several times and this can hinder the build-up of sexual tension. What's important is that you've learnt a lot about your lover's body today and that information will lay the foundation for lots of great sex to come.

Now it's your turn to lie back and allow your lover's fingers do the walking.

Exercise D

Pleasuring Him By Hand (Women Only) – A Guide to Manually Pleasing Men

A lot of women aren't very confident about masturbating their men, understandably, given that all men are proficient masturbators. Many of them feel that if their partners are so well practised in the art, how can they ever compete? But sex isn't a competition – it's a way of sharing an intimate experience, and your hands are capable of producing unique and amazing sensations that your partner could not create alone.

The key ingredient to pleasuring by hand is lubricant. This is particularly important with partners who are circumcised, as the only natural lubrication on the penis – other than pre-ejaculatory fluid (or pre-come, the clear fluid secreted through the urethra prior to ejaculation) – is found beneath the foreskin.

Even in men who aren't circumcised, there's a risk of over-stretching the foreskin when you don't use lube. Plus, dry-hand techniques can also chafe the delicate skin of the penis. Finally, lubricant also allows you to move more fluidly, reducing stress on the muscles and joints in your arm, and allowing you to carry on for far longer than you would with dry hands.

So, before you continue with his arousal massage, apply lots of water-based lubricant to your palms. If you need to reapply lube at any stage, make sure one hand continues to stroke your lover's penis while you use the other to pour lube directly over your working hand.

Perineum and Testicle Massage

In the final stage of the arousal massage (see p. 43), you were stroking your man's mons pubis, or pubic mound; now I'd like you to bring your hands down either side of his penis and testicles to the patch of skin just behind them – the perineum. Using your middle finger, firmly stroke up and down this smooth stretch of flesh. You can even continue further, passing over the anus and moving between his buttocks before bringing your middle finger back up again.

Next, move on to his testicles: gently stroke that middle finger up over the central line, or median raphe of his scrotum, between his testicles, then take one testicle between your finger and thumb and gently roll it.

Real Sex
Two-for-one Hand-job

I can't remember how this came about – it wasn't premeditated in any way. I was kneeling on the bed between my girlfriend's legs. I started to masturbate slowly as she watched, and then she started to play with herself too. Next thing, she'd shuffled down the bed closer to me, so that as I was masturbating, the back of hand – my knuckles – were brushing up and down against her clit too. Best hand-job ever... and very energy-efficient!

Peter, 30

Repeat this move on the other testicle. Ask him how that feels. Some men love it; others can take it or leave it.

Penis Strokes

Just as you were asked to explore your own body on Day One, men were required to do the same. While you continue to massage his perineum and testicles, ask him to show you which strokes turned him on most. As he does so, encourage him by saying how sexy it is to watch him masturbate. If seeing his pumping biceps turns you on, say so. If the look on his face makes you want to sit on it, tell him. The more freely you can speak, the less self-conscious he will feel about touching himself in front of you.

Make a mental note of the position of his hand, how tightly he grips himself, whether the thumb of his fist is positioned on the underside or upper side of his shaft and how far up and down the shaft his hand moves.

Don't let him get too carried away, though. He's meant to be demonstrating his favourite techniques rather than rushing to a 'happy ending'. There's far more to explore before that point.

Now, take his penis in your own well-lubricated fist, and, adopting a similar method to his own, slowly build momentum to establish your basic hand stroke, checking that he's happy with the pressure and pace. Generally men like quite a firm grip – if you're unsure ask him to clasp his hand around your own until the pressure is just right.

Once mastered, you could use this stroke to take him all the way to orgasm, but you can also build far more sexual tension if you extend play with some advanced hand techniques.

Advanced Hand-play Techniques for Him

Special 'extras' are what makes hand stimulation from you so, well, special. Men often masturbate in a perfunctory way, hastily getting from A (for Arousal) to B (for 'Better get a tissue') as quickly possible. It's rare for them to spoil themselves with an erotic and languorous build-up to climax, and that's where your advanced hand-play techniques come in. The following suggestions are designed to inspire you – some he'll love, some he won't. You don't need to try them all today – unless he wants you to – but you should be able to find a few moves that'll make him melt.

- **The basket.** Sit between his legs, then interlock your fingers to form a kind of 'basket' with your hands. Firmly clasp the 'basket' around the base of his penis, then slide it up to the top of his shaft. Next, bring your interlocked fingers all the way over the head of his penis and then back again. Now slide your hands back to the base, and repeat the move continually.

- **The twist.** Again, sit between his legs and grip the base of his penis in your non-dominant hand to steady it. With your dominant hand (palm facing away from you), clasp the base of his penis (just above your steadying hand). Pull your hand to the end of the shaft and – now, here's the complicated bit – twist and turn your fist so it rotates around the head and your palm ends up facing you. It takes a bit of practice to master the twist: your palm will turn through about 180 degrees around the coronal ridge before it then needs to loop over the top of the head. Complicated it may be, but it's precisely all this coronal and head contact that makes the move so spine-tingling for him.

  Next, simply slide your hand down to the base of the shaft and back up to the head where you will repeat the twist in reverse, rotating your fist so your palm now points away from you again. Then go down and back up the shaft as before, continually repeating the move until it becomes one fluid motion.

Extra-curricular Activity
Practice makes perfect

As well as writing books, I run workshops at which I teach women how to perfect hand and oral stimulation. In the classes, my students practise on lifelike dildos with suction bases (secured to plates on a table) or cucumbers held erect between their knees to steady them. This is the ideal way to get to grips with new hand and oral techniques before trying them out on a partner.

- **The pulse.** You may need a little extra lube for this one. Position your full fist around the corona where the shaft and head of his penis meet. Your grip should be quite loose to begin with, but then, while simultaneously moving up the head a fraction, squeeze your fist. Rhythmically repeat this move so it feels like a pulse. Though too subtle for some men, this sensation mimics the feeling of a woman's pubococcygeal (PC) muscles contracting on orgasm, and makes incredibly light work for the arms.

Extra-curricular Activity
Delaying techniques

Changing tempo a few times during any sex session is a good thing – it helps to delay orgasm, allowing more sexual tension to build, and the more tension you have, the more powerful your release (aka orgasm). However, if you change tempo too often you could lose arousal altogether.

For the purposes of this class, you're experimenting with a variety of new techniques, which will automatically create a few changes of tempo. As such, it's unlikely that you'll need to employ delaying techniques. However, if you do, or should you need to in the future, here are two tricks that work:

1. The squeeze. When he's about to tip over the edge, squeeze the head (or glans) of his penis between your thumb and fingers (your thumb should be sitting over his frenulum with your fingers on the top side of his glans). This will force the blood that creates his erection out of the penis and help reduce his arousal almost instantly.

2. The testes tug. Form a hoop around the top of his scrotum and gently pull down, moving his testicles away from his body. When a man ejaculates his testicles travel up towards his body and this reverses that process.

● **The corona hoop.** It may sound like a fifties' dance move, but this is actually far simpler than anything you'd see on a doo-wop dance floor. Create a hoop with your middle finger and thumb (or as close to a hoop as you can get), then rapidly 'bounce' the hoop up and down over his corona.

● **Satin strokes.** You can use items found around the home to enhance masturbation for him. Try wrapping your soft silk or satin knickers around his shaft before you start to masturbate him. The fabric against his flesh will feel luxurious and seeing your lingerie is an added visual arouser.

- **Anal play.** While you're masturbating him, tentatively massage his perineum and then stroke a finger around the circle of his anus. Men who are averse to anal play will generally pull away at this point or move your hand if they don't wish you to go any further. If he doesn't flinch, however, after a few minutes of circling his anus, slide your (well-lubricated) finger inside his bottom – your nails should be clean and neatly trimmed. Wiggle your finger up towards his stomach and a few centimetres inside the rectum, on the front rectal wall, you'll feel a fleshy nub, similar in texture to your own G-spot. This is his prostate and 'milking' it with firm, repetitive 'come-hither' strokes gives some men the most powerful orgasms they can experience. But it's essential to keep masturbating him at the same time, so find a rhythm that's comfortable, allowing you to keep both hands moving simultaneously.

- **Position possible.** As well as experimenting with techniques, try experimenting with positions. Him lying on his back with you between his legs is a good position for some of the more complicated two-hand moves featured above, but you could also try:

  - Sitting to either the left or right of his body, facing his hips as he lies back – this way your hands can easily travel north and south of his waistband, making it a great position to be in if your man likes you to play with his nipples while you masturbate him (a lot of men do!).
  - Lying parallel to him and reaching over his body to his groin – this is the easiest way to emulate his own signature move, as you'll be coming from the same angle.
  - Spooning, with you lying on your side directly behind him – again, a good way to emulate his signature move (if you can reach your hand around far enough).
  - Both of you standing, either facing each other (great for passionate kissing) or with you behind him reaching around – a position that works really well when performed in front of a full-length mirror; just imagine the view!

Well done! You've successfully completed Day Two of *7 Days to Amazing Sex*. You've learnt how to use your hands as sex toys, and now it's time for you to put your talent where your mouth is, as tomorrow you'll be learning how to do the same thing with your tongue!

Day Three
Sex by Mouth

The two key ingredients to giving great oral sex are the right attitude and hot technique; the two key ingredients to *receiving* it are communication and personal preparation. Today, while the intercourse ban still prevails, I'm going to show you how to acquire these keys and unlock the secrets to out-of-this-world oral sex. But first, I'd like you both to create your own personalised erogenous body maps.

Exercise A
Mapping Your Erogenous Zones – Creating a Personalised Body Map of Your Hot Spots

You can use your mouth to pleasure every single inch of your partner's body – not just their genitals. And before you go there, a teasing journey of kisses, licks and sucks will prime your partner, boosting their orgasmic potential. Here are just some of the hot spots on the human anatomy. As you read through these, I'd like you to make a mental note of your own special hot spots, as I'll be asking you about those later.

Real Sex
The Hot Shoulder

My ears, neck and shoulders are the most sensitive parts of my body – after the obvious bits, of course. I know a lot of people like to have their ears nibbled or their necks kissed, but for me the sensitivity stretches all the way across the tops of my shoulders. When a woman kisses me here – or rather kisses, licks, nibbles and sucks here – I get an instant erection. It's not an area many women focus on though, so I have to request it. I always think it makes me sound a bit weird, asking for my shoulders to be kissed, but that's just the way I'm wired. I like what I like.

Jason, 28

- **Lips.** The thin skin of the lips makes them highly sensitive to touch. Try tracing the tip of your tongue around your lover's pout, then gently suck their top and then their bottom lip – Tantric practitioners believe this sends send sex signals straight to the groin. How is it for you?

- **Ears.** Nibble and suck on the lobes, flick your tongue around the surface of the ear, breathe – but *don't* blow – into the ear through either your nose or mouth, making 'Mmmm' sounds as you do so. The sound will send vibrations through the ear and a shiver down the spine.

- **Neck.** The neck is designed to be super sensitive, so we can react quickly to anything that might injure one of our main arteries. This also makes it massively responsive to sexual attention. A passionate French kiss, delicate, light licks with the tip of a pointed tongue or even a (*gentle*) bite here can quickly trigger arousal. But don't ever suck – this creates 'love bite' bruising, which looks ridiculous on teenagers and even worse on adults.

- **Armpits.** Anywhere that's sensitive enough to be ticklish is sensitive enough to respond to sexual touch. Light strokes may trigger giggle fits, but a quick firm lick is strangely pleasant. Also, the armpits – like the crotch – are thought to secrete those pheromones that act as aphrodisiacs on the opposite sex. Research suggests that in women, the 'pherometre' is cranked up to full blast during the most fertile time of their menstrual cycle to help attract a mate, so men planting a few kisses here mid-cycle should remember to inhale.

- **Nipples.** Men as well as women enjoy having their nipples sucked, circled with the tip of a tongue and lightly nibbled. Men should try the 'niptease': trace your tongue around the entire circumference of her breast, moving in ever-decreasing circles to the tip of her nipple – the short wait for you to reach it will be agonising (in a good way).

- **Upper legs.** Peppering both the inner and outer thighs all the way up to the buttocks with wet, sucking kisses, light bites and soft licks will send tingle after tingle to your partner's groin. The thin skin on the back of the knee is also sensitive and deserves a brush with a slow, teasing tongue.

- **Feet.** Ever had your toes sucked? It's the most bizarre experience, and, for me at least, I still can't decide whether it's sexual, soothing or just plain strange. What I do know is that a relatively large area of the brain is reserved for receiving information from your feet, which may explain why they've become revered as sex objects in fetish circles. If your lover is open to having their toes toyed with (and not everybody is) offer a footbath for foreplay (and hygiene reasons!), then try it to see how he or she reacts.

Real Sex
Footsie

As a hairdresser, I'm on my feet all day, and the release I get from a good foot rub does more for my sex life than any back massage ever could. It's like I carry all my tension around in my feet, and when they're firmly massaged all the tension breaks up and starts to melt, then I get waves of pure pleasure travelling all the way up my legs. A foot rub followed by oral sex is my idea of heaven.

Eve, 42

Now, I'd like you to think about all the areas that you really like to have licked, sucked or kissed. Overleaf you'll see two sets of images showing the front and back of both the male and female body. Please mark an 'X' over all the areas you class as erogenous on your own body.

His Hot Spots

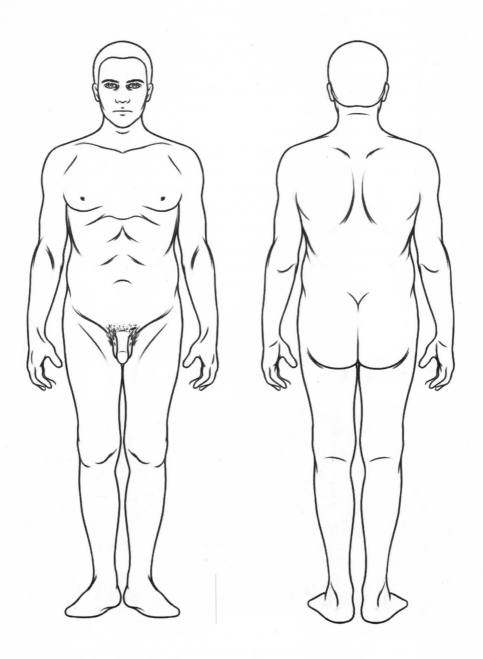

Her Hot Spots

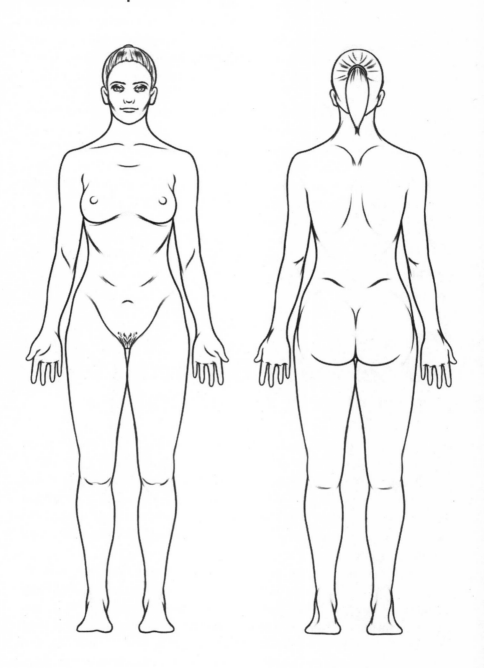

Now that you've successfully completed your erogenous body map, you and your partner both have a crystal-clear picture of where you each like to be kissed, licked and touched. It's essential you leave no erogenous zone unmarked from your fingers to your toes, so check back to make sure you haven't missed any. Were there any surprises that your partner didn't know about? I hope so – this is a journey of sexual discovery, after all.

You can refer back to these maps whenever you need to refresh your memories (and the parts that other lovers don't normally reach!). You can also use a different coloured pen to update your maps at any time. This is useful to do, particularly after an all-over kissing and caressing session, as many people will find their sexual desires shift over time as a result of physical changes, new fantasies or simply boredom from repetition.

Today, you'll each begin your practical oral-sex class by following your lover's maps with your mouths, so bookmark the page. But before we go any further, it's time to prepare for the hottest oral-sex session of your lives.

Exercise B

Oral Sex Prep – The Secrets to Feeling Good About Oral Sex

Lying back while another human being puts their head between your legs is one of the most intimate and also intimidating sex acts many people will ever experience. A lot of us worry about how we appear down there. Have we missed a bit of random loo roll? Is there a stray long head hair stuck between our butt cheeks from the shower we had earlier? Do we look OK? Do we smell OK? Are we wet enough? Dry enough? Small enough? Big enough?

It's understandable that so many people suffer from low genital-esteem – it's the part of our bodies few people ever get to see, including ourselves! I suggested genital-esteem boosting exercises on Day One (self-pleasuring in front of a mirror and creating sexy images of your genitals to gain an appreciation of their sexual appeal – see p. 15), and anyone with issues in this respect should continue to use those exercises. Additionally, there are three steps to preparing for oral sex that will ensure both you and your lover enjoy it to the max:

Step 1: Flattery Gets You Everywhere (Even Down There!)

When was the last time you complimented your lover on their genitals? Regular, positive reinforcement from our lovers helps us to feel good about ourselves, just as negative comments will chip away at our confidence. Telling your partner that you love the way they look, taste and smell will make them more open and receptive to your every touch, so if you want to be really good at oral sex, use that tongue for positive affirmations as much as practical techniques!

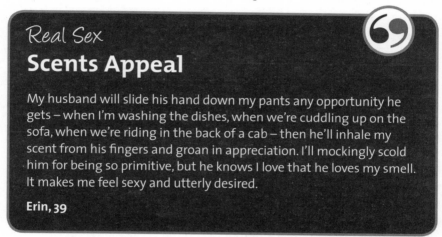

Real Sex
Scents Appeal

My husband will slide his hand down my pants any opportunity he gets – when I'm washing the dishes, when we're cuddling up on the sofa, when we're riding in the back of a cab – then he'll inhale my scent from his fingers and groan in appreciation. I'll mockingly scold him for being so primitive, but he knows I love that he loves my smell. It makes me feel sexy and utterly desired.

Erin, 39

Step 2: Get Fresh

At the same time as complimenting your partner, it's important to take as much pride in your own genital appearance as you would with the way you look overall – and that means freshening up for your lover prior to every oral-sex session. You can either share a cleansing ritual: shower or bathe together, gently washing each other's intimate parts with a flannel or soft natural sponge and warm water. Don't use soap – it can sting and upset the pH balance of the delicate genital skin, which can actually cause funky odours, rather than combat them.

Alternatively, you can freshen up alone. For a quick clean-up, nip to the bathroom and use a non-scented cleansing wipe (such as a baby or feminine hygiene wipe – men can use these too). Or you could soak a flannel in warm water, then wring it out and use it in the same way as a wipe.

Real Sex
Kissed Better

My girlfriend always kisses me after she's given me head – at first, I was a bit grossed out by it because I could taste myself on her lips, but now I actually appreciate the fact that she thinks nothing of kissing me because, to her, there's nothing wrong with how I taste.

Steven, 43

Step 3: Hair Today, Gone Tomorrow?

The debate about pubic hair rages on: is it politically correct to shave down there, or does it reflect some dubious desire for prepubescence? Is it worth the hassle, the regrowth and the resulting irritation? Is it fair that women are expected to do it in a society that's more likely to think of a pubic hairstyle than a South American citizen when they hear the term 'Brazilian'?

It's time for a reality check: politics should be left at the bedroom door, pubic grooming *is* a hassle, but, unfortunately for women, our pubes do tend to get in the way a little more than men's due to our anatomical design, the clitoris being hidden between hair-covered labia, while the head of the penis is a lot further removed from the male thatch.

Some people like a full-haired look, but no one likes the feeling of hair in their mouths. So, there are three options for everyone, regardless of gender, and they are: trim, tug or remove.

- **Trim.** After a bath or shower, if you have a steady hand, *very* carefully trim back pubes using scissors or, better (and safer) still, use an intimate shaver with a gradient guard to prevent cutting the hair too short.

- **Tug.** If you'd rather keep your thatch, prior to oral sex, tug down firmly on your pubes – this will dislodge any loose ones that would otherwise end up stuck between your lover's teeth. Even if you trim your hair, you should still do this prior to oral sex. Try it now and see how many stray hairs you catch – you'll be surprised.

● **Remove.** There are several options for removing all or part of your pubic hair. Salon treatments include waxing, electrolysis and laser hair removal. I've tried them all and know that it's impossible to keep your dignity intact through any of them, so an understanding beautician who you feel comfortable with is essential. The treatments are just about equally painful, and while laser is the most expensive, it is also the most effective in that there are no ingrown hair issues (as there are with waxing), it takes longer for the hair to grow back, and when it does, the hair is finer. After around six treatments, the hair may take months or even years to reappear (as opposed to up to two weeks with waxing) and some people report permanent hair loss. (Though I have to add, that hasn't happened for me after ten treatments.)

In the privacy of your own bathroom, electric shavers and epilators, razors, hair-removal creams and home-waxing kits are your options. The latter, I've never found to work. Electric shaving, epilating and creaming nether regions, all being less than glamorous, are best executed alone with a well-angled mirror.

However, a slow and studied wet shave has erotic overtures that many couples enjoy sharing. Take turns sitting on

Course Notes
Lights on/ lights off?

If you still feel uncomfortable about receiving oral sex and hate doing it with the lights on, despite cleansing and preening your private parts, there's a little trick that may work for you: introduce a blindfold into oral play. The giver can wear the blindfold and you can order them (in a sexily dominant fashion) to use their hands and tongue to feel their way around your genitals. They can't see you, so you're less body-conscious; however, the quality of the oral sex may suffer when your partner is working blind.

Alternatively, you can wear the blindfold. If you're body-conscious you may be wondering how this would work – after all, your partner can still see everything you're desperate to hide. However, it really does work as it helps you to disconnect from all that is visual. For you, it will feel like you're doing it with the lights off and you'll be able to better focus on the sensations while your partner will be able to see exactly what they're doing, making it even better for you.

the edge of the bathtub while your partner sits between your legs and carefully shapes or completely removes your curls, then wash each other down. This makes for a perfect prelude

Extra-curricular Activity
Oral condiments

If you want to add spice to your oral sex life, here are six options:

- **Flavoured lube.** When it comes to oral sex, there's a school of thought that says 'the wetter the better', and once you've tried using flavoured lube for oral sex, it may become a way of life.

  Flavoured lubricants works in two ways: the lubricant itself provides extra fluid, while the sweetness of the lube activates your saliva glands. Additionally, the myriad flavours available, from 'Apple Martini' to 'Chocolate Cherry' (my favourite), offer variety to the giver, and if the taste of genitals doesn't turn you on, they also provide a mask. However, that's the very same reason some people don't like flavoured lube – because the unique taste of a lover can act as a huge aphrodisiac.

- **Popping candy.** The next time you see a packet of popping candy in a store, put it in your basket, then take it home and store it with your sex toys. Then, whenever you want to add some mini explosions to oral sex, sprinkle it on your tongue just before you go down. The sensation is novel rather than mind-blowing, but it brings a sense of fun to the proceedings.

- **Hot drinks.** When asked what makes oral sex feel so great, many people list warmth right up there with wetness, so don't let that cup of bedtime cocoa go to waste. Hold warm fluid in your mouth until your mouth heats up, then swallow the fluid and immediately put your partner in your mouth.

to oral sex, as knowing you're both fuzz-free and fresh makes you feel more comfortable about receiving oral sex as well as giving it.

- **Ice.** Chill thrills aren't for everybody. Ice is generally used to numb sensation, and in sex we'd usually rather embrace it – but if you want to postpone climax, cooling things down can help to prolong play. Also, the contrast of icy coldness followed by heat can sensitise genitals. So, for maximum sensation, suck on an ice cube for a few seconds, then perform oral sex (you can spit out the cube first or keep it in your mouth if it's small and smooth enough), then, after a moment or two, take a warm drink and resume oral sex, continuing to switch for as long as your partner seems interested. (**Note:** *never* place ice directly on to a person's skin before the ice has already begun to melt as it can stick to the skin and cause ice burns.)

- **Champagne.** For this trick to work the champers needs to be chilled and extremely bubbly. You take a mouthful, and, holding it in your mouth, you then suck in your partner's penis or clitoris forming a watertight seal between your lips and their bits so no champagne is lost. The sensation of fizzing bubbles that you feel on your tongue is similar to what they feel on their genitals. You then swallow the champers and continue oral as normal, or repeat the process a few times. The novelty does wear off quite quickly, though (especially if you start slurring your sucks, so to speak), so don't finish the bottle!

- **Mints and mouthwash.** Menthol is often used in lubricants and so-called 'climax creams' as it causes the skin to tingle. Some people find this irritating and uncomfortable, while others find they're more sensitised. You can get the same effect by sucking on a strong mint, or gargling with a strong mouthwash immediately before giving your partner oral sex.

Exercise C

Take Up Your Positions – Discover the Perks of Your Favourite Oral Sex Positions

During oral sex, both giver and receiver need to be physically and mentally comfortable. It helps to choose a position that appeals to your sexual personality (are you more dominant or submissive?), that makes you feel sexy (does you bum look good in this?) and that's sustainable (can you really hold this position until climax?). Fortunately, there are quite a few oral sex positions to choose from.

Together, read the perks of each pose, below, then separately write down the names of the ones you would most like to try without showing each other your answers. Once your lists are complete, compare notes. The ones you both list are the ones to try tonight. If you didn't list any of the same options, negotiate which you'd be prepared to experiment with instead. Keep those that are left over as ways to vary oral sex sessions in future.

Cunnilingus Positions

Try the following:

Missionary

She lies on her back; he can approach from between her legs or he can position himself at her side. Each angle will result in slightly different sensations for her. The question is, which is her favourite? Suck it and see.

- **Her perks:** this stomach-flattening position is flattering; you can look down and enjoy the view or look up at the headboard and lose yourself in fantasy; you can dig your heels into the bed or wrap them around his shoulders to thrust your groin further into his face if he's between your legs; you can play with your breasts or use your hands to part your labia giving him greater access.

● **His perks:** you can switch angles to combat position fatigue (but don't change tempo too often as this could hinder her climax); if you aren't using both arms to lean on, you could play with her breasts – but spare fingers are generally used more effectively for penetration; you can look up and watch her writhe in pleasure, and you have a great view of her genitals.

Hovering butterfly

He lies on his back; she straddles his face so her genitals are hovering over his mouth.

● **Her perks:** you get to control the pace and pressure, but you'll need stamina and will have to be careful not to smother him (unless he's into that sort of thing . . .).

● **His perks:** you feel utterly dominated; your neck will be supported and you can use cushions for added support if needed; you can reach up and play with her bouncing breasts and you can penetrate her anally and vaginally with forefinger and thumb of the same hand (which will also provide a buffer between yourself and suffocation).

Standing

She stands, but to allow greater access to her genitals, it's best if one leg is raised and perched on the edge of a bed or chair that he can also sit on.

● **Her perks:** this will bring out your inner dominatrix, adding a role-play frisson to oral sex.

● **His perks:** you will feel like her sex slave; there's less stress on the neck in this position than in those where she's lying down; you can grip and massage her bum; and you can insert two fingers inside her vagina and make that 'come-hither' motion to stimulate her G-spot, rhythmically pulling her clitoris towards your mouth with each stroke.

Sitting

She sits on the edge of a chair or bed; you kneel between her legs so your face is level with her vulva.

- **Her perks:** once you're sitting comfortably, he can part your thighs with his hands, then slide fingers from both hands up inside your vagina giving you as much fullness as you desire. Who needs ten inches when you have ten digits?

- **His perks:** depending on the dimensions of the furniture available to you, this can be an extremely comfortable position – though don't forget to place a cushion on the floor before kneeling down. She can also use the springs in the bed or chair to bounce herself up and down on your pointed tongue – your tongue doesn't even need to move!

Rear entry

She gets down on all fours; he does the same and licks her from behind in this passionate, animalistic pose.

- **Her perks:** if you like the sensation of having your bottom licked (and millions of us do!), or you like being vaginally penetrated by tongue, this is the position for you. Access to the clitoris may be restricted for him, but you can stroke your clitoris yourself while his tongue works its magic elsewhere.

- **His perks:** while you lick her erogenous zones, you can masturbate yourself at the same time.

Fellatio Positions

Woman on top

He reclines; she kneels between his legs or to the side of his body, bending over to take his penis in her mouth.

Course Notes

Safe anal-oral sex

Bacteria from the anus should never be transferred to the vagina as this can lead to infection. To prevent the spread of harmful bacteria, a man should not move his tongue directly from anus to vagina without using an antibacterial mouthwash in between or placing a latex barrier between his tongue and his lover's bottom and genitals. Dentists use latex squares called dental dams and they're available online, at sex stores and dental supplies stores. You can also cut the head off a condom, slice down one side and unroll it to create a latex square. The latex is then placed over the orifices, so they can be licked through the latex without any spread of bacteria.

- **Her perks:** you can move around his body until you find the position most comfortable for your mouth and his manhood; you can control the pace; you can play with his testicles, massage his perineum or slide a finger inside his anus using one hand, while the other masturbates his shaft in time with your licks and sucks; at certain angles you can make great eye contact.

- **His perks:** you're completely relaxed; you have a great view of the action; and, if she's sitting to the side of your body, you can reach down to play with her bottom and vulva.

Standing

He stands; she kneels before him, her face level with his crotch.

- **Her perks:** with a cushion under your knees this position can be one of the most comfortable positions for giving fellatio; both hands are free to masturbate, penetrate and massage his genitals.

- **His perks:** you'll feel sexually dominant and powerful; it's a great position for eye contact; and it'll feed any porn film fantasies you have, as this is the classic X-rated B-J position. It's also great for 'tea-bagging' (dipping your testicles in her mouth) – but it's equally bad for gagging if you thrust too hard, so let her set the pace.

Sitting

He sits on the edge of a chair or bed; she kneels between his legs.

- **Her perks:** for you, the perks are almost identical to when he stands for oral sex, although you can control his movements more easily, bearing down on his thighs with your arms.

- **His perks:** less tiring than standing, but with the same sexy eye-contact opportunities.

Straddling

This position is exclusively for testicle stimulation. She lies in missionary position; he straddles her body keeping his own upright, moving up her torso until his testicles are level with her mouth.

- **Her perks:** you can masturbate to your heart's content and/or slip a finger inside his anus to massage his G-spot.

- **His perks:** if you like the sensation of dipping your testicles in your partner's mouth, adopt this position and masturbate yourself at the same time for a truly explosive sensation.

The deep-throat trick

She lies back on a bed with her head hanging over the edge, thus straightening and elongating her throat, making it 'deeper'; he kneels in front of her, bringing his penis level with her open mouth, and enters gradually and slowly.

- **Her perks:** you get to do 'deep throat' without gagging; he can play with your nipples and you can masturbate yourself at the same time.

- **His perks:** you get to say you've experienced the much sought-after 'deep throat' – but don't expect too much. As you well know, the majority of nerve endings are in the head of your penis and when it's down the back of her throat she can't do all those wonderful swirling and flicking actions with the tip of her tongue.

Reciprocal Positions

Reciprocal oral-sex positions – most commonly referred to as '69' because of the reversed shape of the numbers (or 'soixante-neuf', because everything sounds a little sexier in French) – are fun to experiment with, but because it's difficult to focus on receiving pleasure while you're giving it, few couples can climax this way. However, that doesn't stop this kinky oral sex position from being a good starting point to any session. Here are the classic configurations to try:

Man on top

She lies in missionary position; he straddles her face, bending forwards to bring his face in line with her genitals.

- **Her perks:** you're in the most comfortable reclined position, and, rather than taking his penis directly into your mouth, you can masturbate him while flicking your tongue over the head, which will also prevent him over-thrusting into your throat.

● **His perks:** you get to lick her clitoris from a totally new angle, but remember to place your fingers on her pubic mound and pull back towards you, as this will also pull back the clitoral hood giving your tongue greater access.

Woman on top

He lies flat on his back; she straddles his face, bending forwards, so her mouth is in line with his penis.

● **Her perks:** you control the pace and depth at which you take him in your mouth, as well as being able to thrust against his tongue.

● **His perks:** being the reclining partner, you're able to relax more; you can also reach down and feel her breasts swinging as she bounces against you.

Side by side

Both partners lie on their sides, torsos slightly raised on their lower arms, facing the other's genitals; she bends her knee and lifts her upper leg, resting the foot just behind her lower leg to allow him greater access.

● **His 'n' her perks:** this is the most mutually comfortable of the reciprocal oral sex positions; both partners can equally control pace.

Now, reveal to each other which oral sex positions you'd most like to try, then get ready for your practical. Decide who will be first to be the receiver, refer back to your respective erogenous body maps to plan your course of kisses, then, ladies, read on for some hot tips for tongue play, and men, turn to page 77 for your Mouth Muscle Masterclass.

Course Notes
Sex furniture

When creating a space for oral sex, it's advisable to dot around as many pouffes and cushions as possible; these can be used to elevate body parts for easier access or simply to support them to combat fatigue. A cleverly positioned, plump pillow can make the difference between average and out-of-this-world orgasmic oral sex.

Exercise D

Hot Tips on Tongue Play (Women Only) – Fellatio Tricks that Every Woman Should Know

In the final part of today's class, it's time to get your tongue around some hot techniques, but before you do, let's have a quick word about the spit/swallow debate. Some women either enjoy, or at least don't mind, the taste of semen and swallowing it isn't an issue for them. That's fine, so long as it's safe to exchange bodily fluids with your partner. It's generally considered safe when a couple has been monogamous for at least six months following previous sexual encounters with other people and then had full STI tests (this allows enough time for infections to be detected). If you aren't in that situation, swallowing is a very bad idea, and using condoms (preferably flavoured ones) for oral sex is advisable.

If you would rather not swallow, that's fine too. You should enjoy giving oral sex as much as your partner enjoys receiving it – and if you don't, it's unlikely that he'll enjoy it at all. Remember what you've already learnt today: the right attitude is one of the key ingredients to being able to give your lover hot oral pleasure.

Women who aren't keen on the taste of semen can use flavoured lubes to mask and dilute the taste, and/or take the penis further into their throat at the point of orgasm – as most taste buds are towards the front of the tongue, the further back the semen hits, the less flavour there'll be. You can also try suggesting a fruitier diet for your man as strawberries and pineapples sweeten the taste of semen, while alcohol and spicy food such as curries are best avoided. Alternatively, take the seriously sexy option of allowing him to ejaculate over a part of your body instead (face, breasts and bottom being the most popular options with guys).

The one thing you should never do is a series of facial contortions as you spit out his semen. Imagine how you would feel if a man who had been going down on you started to do the same. Decide in advance how you'd like to handle his climax, and then enjoy every moment.

Now that's cleared up, let the fun begin.

Step 1: Demo Time

Before going down on your man, slide your fingers in his mouth. Then, in your sexiest voice, ask him to suck, lick and kiss them exactly how he would like you to suck, lick and kiss his penis. You can masturbate him with your free hand while he does his demo, then repeat his moves, or you can copy the moves in real time. The latter requires more concentration, but is guaranteed to make him melt, as this is the closest most men will ever get to giving themselves oral sex.

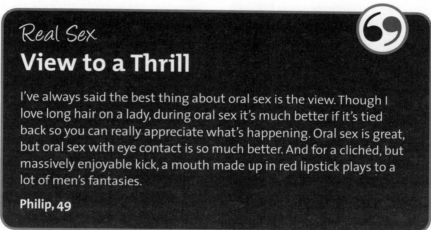

Real Sex
View to a Thrill

I've always said the best thing about oral sex is the view. Though I love long hair on a lady, during oral sex it's much better if it's tied back so you can really appreciate what's happening. Oral sex is great, but oral sex with eye contact is so much better. And for a clichéd, but massively enjoyable kick, a mouth made up in red lipstick plays to a lot of men's fantasies.

Philip, 49

Step 2: Hand-to-Mouth Co-ordination

Fellatio without hands is like cake without cream. On Day Two of my plan you learnt how to use your hands as sexual tools, and that talent will be vital in making your fellatio skills legendary (in your own bedroom at least!). Your hands can also take the 'job' out of B-Js, making fellatio easy and enjoyable. Here's how:

- **The ring.** Firmly gripping the base of your man's member will steady his penis and help to keep blood locked in his erection, making him harder and more sensitive to your touch. Your hand can also act as a stopper, preventing him from thrusting further into your mouth than you would like.

- **Basic masturbation.** While your tongue focuses on the head of his penis, always massage the shaft in his preferred hand-job style.

- **Mound massage.** The fleshy pubic mound that protects his pubic bone is responsive to sexual touch, but often neglected. Try firmly circling a thumb from one hand over it while your other hand works his penis.

Real Sex
Lip Gloss

The prettiest thing I ever saw a woman do was take a dab of clear, shiny pre-come from the end of my cock and rub and it around her lips like it was lipstick – I thought I'd died and gone to heaven.

Ben, 22

- **Testicle massage.** Some men enjoy the feeling of having their testicles gently rolled between finger and thumb during oral sex.
- **Perineum massage.** Firmly stroke the patch of skin between his testicles and anus in a 'come-hither' or circular motion.
- **Nipple play.** Reach up and tweak his nipples with your free hand, while your other continues to work his penis. Not all men claim to be sensitive in this area, but by playing with his nipples during other sexual activity you can condition them (or any other nerve-packed part of the body, for that matter) to associate stimulation with arousal. The Russian Noble Prize winner Ivan Pavlov mastered classic conditioning with dogs by producing food, which made the dogs salivate, at the same time as ringing a bell – eventually the sound of the bell alone made the dogs salivate. This is not to suggest that men are dogs, but I have tried this trick and it really does work.
- **Penetration.** You can also slide a well-lubricated finger inside his bottom, firmly and rhythmically pulsing it forwards (towards his stomach) to massage his G-spot – but don't attempt this without asking permission first.
- **The stop-gap stroke.** When your mouth is feeling tired, it's OK to take a break, but continue to masturbate him at the same pace, focusing on the head of his penis where your mouth has

been – this way his climax won't lose momentum, undoing all your efforts.

> ### Extra-curricular Activity
> # How to stop him grabbing your head
>
>
>
> If your man has an uncontrollable tendency to grab your head during oral sex, making the experience uncomfortable for you, tie his hands above his head or behind his back for a simple, yet incredibly sexy solution.

Step 3: Hot Fellatio Techniques

You can use the following techniques in the order they appear for the ultimate oral workout, or you can pick 'n' mix those you'd like to try, adapting them in any way you wish. Add any new moves you devise to the end of the list and keep the book handy, so you can bone up on ideas whenever you want to vary your fellatio format in future.

> ### Real Sex
> # U-spot
>
>
>
> The opening in the end of my penis is really sensitive. When my girlfriend gives me head she dips the very tip of her tongue into it and then flaps her tongue across the top of it really quickly between taking me in her mouth – other than coming, that's the sensation I most enjoy during oral.
>
> **Neil, 31**

- **Tea-bagging.** As a prelude to penis play, gently circle the tip of your tongue around each of his testicles. If he doesn't flinch (some men are extremely protective of their testicles), try a wide, flat lick up through the centre of his scrotum, which is a particularly sensitive spot for a lot of guys. Next, very delicately suck in one testicle and roll your tongue around it before releasing it and repeating the move on the other one.

- **The cob.** Hold his penis between your finger and thumb at the base, then wrap your lips around the left side of the shaft, just above the base. Next, slide your mouth up the shaft, then over the top of the head, letting your tongue swirl around the tip, before sliding your mouth back down the right side of the shaft to the base. Repeat this move going from right to left, then left to right again, and so on, always focusing extra attention on the head – as the majority of nerve endings are contained here, his body will be on edge waiting for you to get back to it, making this a great teasing stroke to warm up with.

- **The swirl.** While masturbating the shaft of his penis, swirl your tongue all the way around the head in one continuous circle. Doing this with deliberate slowness, while making direct eye contact with him, is a hot way to prepare his body and brain for what's about to come (him – hopefully!).

Real Sex
Porn Star

My husband used to come through oral sex in around three to five minutes, but as we've grown older, it can take anywhere between fifteen and twenty – not that I'm counting. It's just that it can be a real strain on my jaw. So, to try to keep up momentum, I fantasise that I'm a porn star being filmed by a room full of cameramen. The idea turns me on and helps to keep me in the moment.

Terri, 42

- **The frenulum flick.** Continuing to masturbate him, rapidly flick your tongue back and forth over the string of skin that attaches foreskin to shaft (or, if he's circumcised, the ridged underside of the head of his penis). You can flick your tongue from side to side or up and down; you can also tilt your head sideways or upright to vary the angle of your tongue flick against his skin – whatever's easier for you.

- **The deep-throat effect.** Wrap your lips around the head of his penis, then wrap your hand around the shaft, so that your hand forms a seal with your mouth – this creates a long, hot flesh tunnel from hand to mouth to give him the sensation of deeper penetration. Then, breathing through your nose, masturbate him with your mouth, following your hand all the way.

List your own hot fellatio techniques here:

_____

_____

_____

_____

Congratulations, ladies – you've completed Day Three of *7 Days to Amazing Sex*, and, no doubt, blown your man's mind in the process! Now, to celebrate, lie back and see just how much he's learnt so far.

Exercise E

Mouth Muscle Masterclass (Men Only) – Oral Sex Skills that Every Man Should Have

Personally, I like a very fast side-to-side tongue stroke directly on the clitoris, with no contact at all at the point of orgasm. If only all women were the same, this exercise would end here. However, we're not – and what's more, no woman's sexual cravings are set in stone. So, some days I feel like having oral sex; others I don't. Also, if oral sex followed the exact-same format described above for the rest of my life, no matter how effective it is right now, I'd soon get bored.

In this exercise you'll learn everything you need to know to give your lover amazing oral sex, but it's up to you to keep it amazing by varying your techniques from time to time. When your partner loves your signature moves, you may be tempted to think, 'If it ain't broke, don't fix it', but sexual boredom is a libido-killer, so it's shrewd to stay one step ahead of it. I'm not talking about scrapping your signature moves and starting from scratch; I'm simply suggesting you include a different warm-up move, introduce a new prop or toy (more on those in Day Five) or flip positions every now and then to maintain a delicious air of unpredictability. Her libido will thank you for it.

And now, it's time for a quick demo.

Step 1: Demo Time

Sit facing your partner, then hold out your palm to her with straight fingers parted between the middle and ring fingers to create a gap (think of the *Star Trek* salute, but with palm facing up). Now place your other hand beneath it and poke your index finger through the gap near the crux of the outstretched fingers. Look and see what you've created. Your outstretched fingers represent labia, while the index finger poking through from beneath represents the clitoris.

Ask your lover to demonstrate on your palm exactly how she likes her labia, clitoris and vagina to be licked. Don't worry if either or both of you get a fit of the giggles – sex and laughter go well together and this is an amazing insight into what your lover really wants.

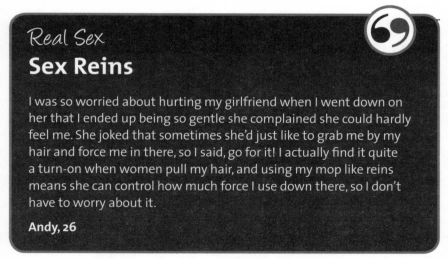

Real Sex
Sex Reins

I was so worried about hurting my girlfriend when I went down on her that I ended up being so gentle she complained she could hardly feel me. She joked that sometimes she'd just like to grab me by my hair and force me in there, so I said, go for it! I actually find it quite a turn-on when women pull my hair, and using my mop like reins means she can control how much force I use down there, so I don't have to worry about it.

Andy, 26

Step 2: Hand-to-Mouth Co-ordination

Think back to the last time you gave a woman oral sex. Visualise the moment. Can you picture the scene? Where were your hands? If they were idle – maybe just cupping her bottom, for example – then you were missing a trick! Hand-to-mouth co-ordination is one of the most important oral sex techniques you'll ever learn and it can mean the difference between forgettable oral sex and fireworks. Here are some moves you can make with your hands to maximise the impact of your tongue techniques:

- **Pube pulling.** This can be sexually arousing in itself, when it's done firmly but not too aggressively. The key is to grip lots of hair at once, so you're moving the flesh with the hair, rather than plucking at a few strands, which just stings. Try gripping a handful of hair on her pubic mound and pull up towards her stomach – this will lift her clitoral hood, exposing her clitoris to more direct touch.

- **Pushing mound.** If hair pulling doesn't excite your partner, use the heel of your hand to push up her pubic mound – this will have the same effect, helping to retract her clitoral hood and expose her clitoris.

- **Parting labia.** Use both hands, or your index and forefinger from one hand to part her outer labia, allowing your tongue greater access to her vagina, urethra, inner labia and clitoris.

- **Breast play.** While one hand and your tongue are working her genitals, use your other hand to explore her body. Simultaneously stroking her breasts and gently pulling at her nipples will send sensations all around her torso for a full-body orgasm, rather than localising all sensation between her legs.

- **Penetration.** While stimulating her clitoris with your tongue, you can simultaneously penetrate her either vaginally or anally (or both!). Remember, though – never transfer fingers (or tongue) directly from anus to vagina as the transfer of bacteria can cause infection. While your fingers are inside her, try adding further digits to give her a more intense fullness; you can thrust fingers to mimic penile penetration, circle your fingers to mimic the rotating shaft of the iconic Rabbit vibrator, or you can use the 'come-hither' finger wiggle for G-spot stimulation.

Step 3: Hot Lady-licking Techniques

The following techniques are designed to inspire – vary them in any way that turns her on and add your own creations at the end of this list. You can then refer back to it as bedtime reading whenever you feel a rut coming on.

- **The long lick.** This is a great way to start any oral-sex session. She lies in missionary position; you lie between her legs, then, with a wide, flat tongue, you slowly lick from just beneath her vaginal opening all the way up to above her clitoris. Three to five of these strokes make powerful teasers, opening her up to more focused clitoral attention.

- **The sucker.** Place your lips around her clitoris to form a seal and gently suck it up and release repeatedly. This envelops the clitoris in warmth and draws blood into it to sensitise it further. For some women, it's a hot warm-up move and for others it's divine at the point of climax if you follow the tempo of her own orgasmic muscular contractions (if your fingers are inside her you'll feel when the pelvic muscles pulse).

Real Sex
Stamina – It's All in the Mind

I love going down on women, but some women want a lot longer than others and if I'm starting to flag, I have to fantasise. The scenarios vary. At the moment I like going down on Angelina Jolie, but it used to be Jennifer Aniston. I guess me and Brad must have similar taste.

Marco, 34

- **The lick-through.** If your lover has an extremely sensitive clitoris, she'll love this move. Rather than tearing off her pants, lick her through the fabric. This is also a great way to tease any woman, especially when you occasionally slip your tongue under her knickers elastic for some flesh-on-flesh contact.

- **The poke**. Poke out your tongue, so it's stiff, then use it as you would a penis to penetrate her. Some women enjoy the novel sensation; others think, 'Why bother penetrating me with two inches of tongue when you have six inches of penis in your pants?' – it's up to your partner to let you know which side of the fence she falls on.

● **Tongue-8.** Moving the tip of your tongue in a figure of eight across her genitals ensures that you circle her clitoris and vagina, while crossing hot spots like the urethra and inner labia along the way. Some people even suggest writing out the alphabet with the tip of your tongue. Personally, I find this a little odd – like being with someone who's distracting himself from his enjoyment by reciting the alphabet – plus, it's difficult to hit upon a rhythm while following the lines of different letters, but if it works for your partner, spell away.

● **The flat no.** Push out your tongue, and then curl it down so it's flat, wide and soft, rather than pointed and firm. Place the flat surface of your tongue against her clitoris, then shake your head from side to side like you're vehemently gesturing, 'No'. This takes pressure off your tongue muscle and allows you to move quickly across her clitoris with as much pressure as she desires.

● **The clit flick.** Part her labia with two fingers to fully expose her clitoris, then flick your pointed tongue over its head. While some women will like the flick to go from side to side, others will prefer it to go up and down over the clitoris. Experiment with both and ask which feels best. If your tongue finds it easier to go one way rather than the other, tilt your head or alter your position accordingly.

List your own cunnilingus creations here:

_____

_____

_____

_____

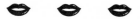

You should now be feeling very happy with yourself. You've successfully completed Day Three of *7 Days to Amazing Sex* – well done! On Day

Four, you'll master the art of intercourse – yes, that means you can finally have full penetrative sex. And, I assure you, it will have been worth the wait.

Day Four
Intelligent Intercourse

You could be forgiven for thinking that women don't enjoy intercourse. Barely a month goes by without a fresh set of statistics landing on my desk reinforcing this persistent rumour. And maybe it's true that only around 30 per cent of women can climax through penetration alone. Frankly, with the clitoris being positioned *outside* of the vagina, it's a miracle that any of us can climax through penetrative sex at all without a little extra assistance. But, the good news is that we don't have to.

To make penetrative sex orgasmic for both parties, all that's required is a vibrator or a helping hand (his or hers, either will do) and possibly a few minor adjustments to your thrusting technique, attitude and/or choice of positions. Today, you're going to learn how to make it happen as you're finally allowed to go all the way.

Exercise A

Position Pick 'n' Mix – Hot Sex Positions For You to Try Tonight

Let's start with the basics. Fundamentally, all sex positions – no matter how kinky or twisted – are variations of the following five moves: man on top, woman on top, rear entry, side by side and standing.

Below, I've listed the classic version of each, plus the perks, followed by a variant you might enjoy. We all have our favourites, but I'd like you to read the notes on all of the positions, noting how you can make each move that little bit hotter, then select four that you'd like to try today. Yes, *four*!

Four position changes during one session is a lot by anyone's quota, but this isn't your average sex session: it's about breaking away from old habits and learning new techniques, even if it involves falling down laughing at some point. And, OK – if you only manage three positions, I'll still be proud of you.

For an element of surprise, you could even write the names of the positions on ten separate pieces of paper, then fold up the papers and place them all in a bowl by your bed – let's call it your Bedside Super Bowl in the spirit of the game. Then, each of you randomly select two pieces of paper and agree to try out whatever positions you find after you've completed today's exercises.

Real Sex

Lube-fall

I love lube – wouldn't have sex without it – and my signature sex move depends on it. When I'm on top of a man, straddling him, I pour lube straight from the bottle over my breasts, focusing on my nipples. You need to use quite a lot to get the waterfall effect. Then I stroke it into my boobs and down my abdomen. It trickles down and covers the guy's pubic bone area and my clit, and once I've massaged it into his stomach and chest, then, and only then do I start grinding.

Maria, 28

Real Sex
Hotdog

A position that works for both me and my hubby doesn't actually involve penetration at all. I straddle him in the usual woman-on-top position – only his erection is lying flat against his abdomen rather than inside me. I pour on my favourite lube like ketchup on his 'hotdog' and then, with my vaginal lips around him, I slide up and down it so my clitoris is rubbing over the head until I climax.

Linda, 38

Man on top

Classic: missionary. She lies on her back, legs parted, knees slightly bent; he lies on top of her with his legs between hers. This is a popular position because it allows maximum skin-on-skin contact, eye contact and kissing. It's also just as good for anal sex as it is for vaginal sex.

- **Her perks:** his pubic bone can grind against your clitoris, or, if he raises his torso up on his arms, you can reach down to masturbate with a hand or toy while he thrusts. For deeper penetration, you can bend one or both of your knees up towards your chest or place a pillow or two beneath your bottom. You can also grab his bottom or wrap your legs around him and dig your heels into it to drive him further into you.

- **His perks:** being on top you have more control of the pace, so make sure you get feedback from her on what feels good. If you can see her clitoris, it means nothing is grinding into it, which is probably a bad sign. Try to align your pubic bone with her clitoris or ask her to play with herself as a visual treat for you. When your torso is raised, she can also play with your nipples.

Variant: coital alignment technique (CAT). From standard missionary position, with him lying directly on top of her, torso to torso, he moves a few inches up his partner's body while his penis is inside her. This pulls his genitals up against hers so he has greater contact with her clitoris. Rather than plunging in and out, he then pushes down with his pelvis and she responds by pushing up with hers to create a repetitive rocking motion.

Some couples swear by this, others can never quite get it right. Try it and see which category you fall into. But remember, you should attempt every new sex move at least twice because what feels awkward one day might just fall into place the next. Think of it as learning to ride a bike: if we all gave up after the first time we fell off there'd be no cyclists on the roads.

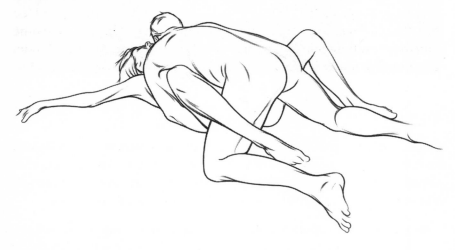

Woman on top

Classic: cowgirl. According to a recent global sex survey by global condom manufacturers Durex, 29 per cent of people prefer woman-on-top positions, making them the world's favourite, and it's understandable why. In the classic cowgirl stance he lies on his back and she straddles him, sitting upright, her legs bent at the knee either side of his body. She can raise her body up and down his shaft, or she can rock her body back and forth, so she's almost sliding up and down his shaft instead (which is easier on the leg muscles and more effective for the clitoris).

● **Her perks:** you control the pace and can make sure your clitoris is getting maximum pubic bone contact by angling your body forwards, or you can lean back and masturbate yourself, while rocking back and forth with the tip of his penis pushing against the front wall of your vagina inside you (hello G-spot!). You can also reach behind you and play with his testicles.

- **His perks:** to help control the pace, you can grab her hips and push her back and forth over your groin. When she's upright or leaning back you have access to her clitoris – use it! If she's leaning forwards, you can suck or play with her nipples too.

Variant: seated embrace. This is a popular Tantric position. From classic cowgirl pose, he sits up, then she wraps her legs around his waist with his penis still inside her; he then crosses his legs beneath her bottom and she rocks in his lap, clenching her pelvic muscles with each move. Kissing and eye contact are key, and you can use co-ordinated deep-breathing exercises to help clear your mind of everything but each other and the sensations you're sharing. At the same time, he can reach around and finger or stroke her bottom to mix the spirituality with a bit of kink.

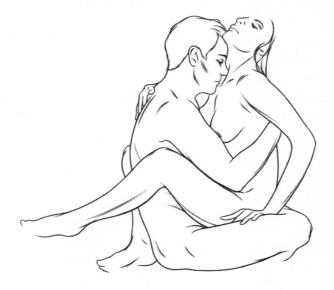

Rear entry

Classic: doggy-style. In the classic rear-entry pose, she positions herself on all fours; he kneels behind her and enters her from behind. These positions work well for both anal and vaginal penetration.

- **Her perks:** you can increase the bend in your knees, lifting your bottom up higher, to increase the depth of his stroke; and you can simultaneously slide a finger inside yourself while he thrusts, for a greater feeling of fullness. You can stroke your clitoris with your hand or toy, or he can reach round and masturbate you; he can also lean forwards to cup and stroke your breasts.

- **His perks:** in addition to the beautiful view of her rear, you get to watch yourself slide in and out of your lover; you can also spank her at the same time, which draws blood to the skin's surface, sensitising it (some women won't thank you for living out that porn-film cliché, but others love it). Or you can slip a finger or toy inside her bottom at the same time to give her 'DP' (double penetration) thrills without having to share her with a second man.

Variant: hot pancakes. So called because you're stacked. She lies flat on her front; he lies on top of her, the full length of his body touching hers. This lessens the depth of rear-entry penetration, making it more comfortable for some women, though for clitoral stimulation a vibe or pillow needs to be strategically placed beneath her (for women who first learnt to masturbate by thrusting into a pillow the action will be second nature). With both parties thrusting down, he nibbles her neck and ears and kneads her breasts.

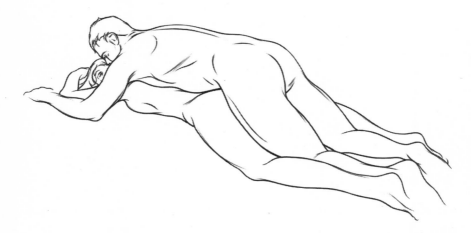

Side by side

Classic: crab embrace. In this side-by-side embrace, the couple lie facing each other: her upper leg goes over his hip, he then shuffles forwards into a comfortable position and penetrates her. Cuddling, kissing and face stroking are also on offer in this relaxed, intimate pose.

● **Her perks:** you can reach down between your legs and masturbate by hand or vibe. The support of a bed under your abdomen also makes this a good position to use during pregnancy.

● **His perks:** you can lick, suck or caress her breasts and you can reach around her body to stimulate her bottom. Penetration may be shallower than with other positions due to the distance between your groins, but this means the head of your penis gets a lot of attention with each stroke. It's also a good position for any man who's a little too well endowed for his partner.

Variant: the mast. From the crab embrace he raises her leg straight up into the air, exposing more of her genitals. This makes the pose feel less romantic and more 'naughty' – it can also allow for greater clitoral access for vibrators and hand play for her.

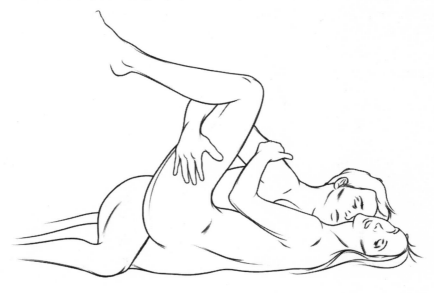

Standing

Classic: up against a wall. Only 2 per cent of the Durex sex survey respondents listed standing sex positions as their favourites; however, that does show that even the most awkward sex positions have their admirers. To try it, she leans back against a wall for balance and support, legs apart; he stands between her legs and enters her, raising one of her legs with his hand to gain easier access.

● **Her perks:** you can stand on stairs and use a handrail for balance if mismatched height is an issue – and hey, at least it drags sex out of the bedroom for a change. Once mastered, standing sex is great for 'on location' quickies, anywhere – from the shower to shop changing rooms – and any time you dare.

● **His perks:** you can dip your head and bury it in her chest. Also, no one will expect anything more than a quickie from you in this position, so premature ejaculation worries are banished.

Variant: the hold. This pose will be quicker still, but it does come in handy if she's much shorter than him. He lifts her in his arms, supporting her with his hands beneath her bottom; she wraps her legs around his hips and her arms around his shoulders. Now for the tricky bit: holding her in one arm (with her gripping him to take as much of her own weight as possible), he uses his other hand to guide himself inside her. Once inserted, she bounces in his arms. Quick, passionate and a great way for him to work out his biceps. (See, I told you sex was good for the figure.)

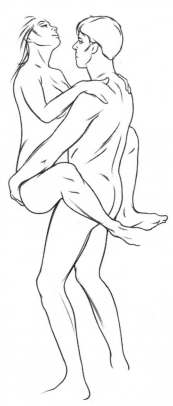

Real Sex
Dry Run

One of the sexiest moments I recall from when I first started dating my girlfriend was a heavy petting session that turned into sex with our clothes on. I was rock-hard beneath my jeans and she – also still fully clothed – was on top of me, cowgirl-style, riding up and down me as though her life depended on it. She came – I was really close, but holding back in case she thought I was a loser for coming in my pants – and then we fell about laughing afterwards, shocked at ourselves for acting like teenagers. I think people should act like teenagers more often.

Cameron, 31

Exercise B
Develop Your Own Sex Position – Just How Creative Are You in Bed?

This next exercise is for fun. Having identified the five basic sex positions and how each can be adapted to create others, I'd like you to work separately and create your own – one that you think will work for you. No conferring. Include whatever props and toys may be necessary to execute the position, and be entirely selfish – sometimes it's OK to be a bit 'Me, me, me'! To help you, consider the following questions:

- What position do you feel most sexy in?
- What's your favourite view during intercourse?
- Is eye contact essential to your arousal?
- Are you more sexually dominant or submissive?
- Do you need to allow room for a prop, such as a vibrator or a pillow?

And, most importantly:

● Which parts of your body need to have physical stimulation in order for you to be able to climax?

Jot down your ideas on a piece of paper (you can even draw a little picture if you're feeling artistic), then show it to your lover and describe how you think it will work.

Though this exercise should raise a few giggles, there's a serious underlying benefit to it because in creating and describing a position that will work for you, you get to show your partner everything you need during intercourse.

Now, you can either use the positions you've created as part of the four you will try out later, or you can add them to your Bedside Super Bowl (see p. 84) and keep the bowl by your bed for extra-curricular games of position pick 'n' mix whenever the fancy strikes.

Course Notes
Anal intercourse

Working girl and author Belle du Jour once said: 'I know anal sex is the new black because my bloody mother just rang up to talk about it.' According to a recent sex survey, 35 per cent of people now indulge, and with so many people doing it, there's more pressure on the rest of us to try it. The question is: do you really want to? Anal sex is unique and thrilling, but it's not for everyone.

If you're female and you'd like to try anal sex with your partner, I recommend that you attempt anal masturbation alone first, as outlined on Day One of my plan (see p. 28). You can use your finger or a specially designed toy (you'll learn more about those on Day Five, see pp. 115–131), and if you enjoy it alone, you're likely to enjoy it with your man, too. Unlike the vagina, the rectum doesn't produce its own natural lubrication so additional lube is essential.

Also, bear in mind that when introducing anything to the anus, the muscles will automatically contract at first, so allow them to relax before letting your man proceed. Opt for a slow and steady thrust and make sure you have some form of clitoral stimulation at the same time.

Anal sex is the easiest way to pass on an STI, so always use a condom unless you're 100 per cent sure of your own and your partner's sexual health. Even then, condoms make anal sex more hygienic, as cleaning up is as simple as throwing away the condom afterwards. Once the condom is discarded, you can go on to have vaginal sex with a fresh one (if you use them for vaginal sex), but – at the risk of sounding repetitive – you must not insert a penis into a vagina after it's been in a bottom unprotected without washing it first as this can spread infection-causing germs.

Extra-curricular Activity
Create your own *Kama Sutra*

A cute way to keep positions fresh is to draw inspiration from the world around you. X-rated or even mainstream films, works of art, porn sites, magazines and sex chats with friends may all throw up ideas. When you discover a position you'd like to try, make a written note of it, or, better still, act it out with your partner and take a Polaroid or digital photo that you can print out. Keep all the images in a scrap book for future reference and, before long, you'll have your very own, very kinky, personalised *Kama Sutra* that you can keep for ever.

Exercise C
Thrusting Styles – Exploring the Ins and Outs of Intercourse

It's not only the positions you have sex in, but also how you thrust against each other that will determine whether intercourse is mutually orgasmic. Here's a selection of thrusting techniques – during your practice session, I'd like you to try using all of them to see which ones work for you as a couple.

- **Pistoning.** Long, deep thrusts – slow or fast – seem to be popular with men. It's how they do it in porn films, and the vision of watching a penis slide inside a vagina is a huge turn-on for both parties. The trouble with this thrust, however, is that the penis can slide all the way out between strokes, making sex clumsy, or worse, leading to the, 'Sorry, I slipped', anal breaking-and-entering routine. When the penis does slide all the way out, then back in again, air can be forced inside the vagina and what goes in must come out, leading to embarrassing sound effects from below. Also, more crucially, the more time the pubic bone spends away from the clitoris, the less likely the woman is to be stimulated. Pistoning has its place: a few long, slow thrusts is a delicious way to start a session, and women who like to feel impact on their cervix are candidates for this move, but men should be aware of its pros and cons before pistoning on regardless. As a general rule of thumb, techniques used in porn films cater to camera angles, not climaxes.

- **Shallow thrusts**. Short, shallow thrusts can be effective for both parties. When the penis is fully inserted, the repeated bouncing of the man's pubic bone against the clitoris, twinned with the internal sensations, may just be enough to make a woman climax in positions where the lovers are facing one another. Men can also try inserting their penis to just below the head and performing shallow thrusts within the first eight or so centimetres of the vagina. This is the tightest part of the vagina, with the greatest concentration of nerve endings, and in forward-facing positions, the head of the penis will be bumping over the woman's G-spot, so both parties could benefit – but only if there is an additional source of clitoral stimulation.

Extra-curricular Activity

Sex décor

You can buy sex furniture to take lovemaking to new heights – literally. Sex swings, which are fitted to supporting beams in ceilings (try explaining that job to your local joiner) make standing positions easy. You can also buy inflatable sex chairs and sofas with dildo seats attached, and upholstered foam wedges that look like funky pouffes in dramatic, angular shapes, allowing you to tip and tilt your bodies into new positions. All are available from sex shops. If you don't have the space or budget, try using your own furniture in inventive ways. A garden swing is great for alfresco frolics at night, when the neighbours can't see over the fence; a footstool could become a bench to lean over during rear-entry scenarios; pillows can elevate body parts to great heights; and we've all heard just how much fun the humble washing machine can be ...

- **Swivelling.** When the penis is fully inserted, rather than thrusting, a man on top can swivel his hips in a circle for an entirely unique and novel sensation, and when a woman is on top she can do the same. This grinding move strokes the clitoris with every rotation, but, as it's difficult to pick up pace, it may not be the best climax clincher for those who require fast strokes.

- **Rocking.** With the penis fully inserted, rather than adopting an in/out motion, a couple actually slide against one another: when the woman is on top, the man can guide her by her hips, pushing her up and down over his groin, and she can grab his shoulders or the headboard and pull herself up and down; when the man is on top, he moves his pelvis up and down, rather than pulling away and then pushing forwards, and the woman can grab his hips or bum and move him up and down between her legs. Contact with the clitoris is constant, the opening to the vagina is being stimulated and penetration is at its deepest, making this an all-round winner.

Exercise D

The Intercourse Troubleshooter – Banishing Bedroom Issues

Just about every couple has issues when it comes to intercourse, unless they're in the hormone-fuelled honeymoon phase – and even then, they aren't exempt. In your final exercise today, I'd like you to identify what's holding back your (penetrative) sex life, then read on for the solution.

The Issue: You Can't Come During Intercourse

This issue tends to affect more women than men, due to the fact that the clitoris doesn't always get much friction during penetrative sex. However, that's not to say that men don't suffer with this problem too. They do, and the same solution applies.

If you're able to orgasm through other means, such as masturbation, you need to apply the same principles of those activities to intercourse.

Just as a woman may only be able to climax if she uses a firm hand stroke or a vibrator on her clitoris, a man may need a *really* firm grip – the sort of grip that not even a vagina that's never passed a baby or missed a pelvic-floor workout can achieve.

While it's easy for a woman to apply a hand or vibe to her clitoris during intercourse due to its location (see, every cloud has a silver lining – take full advantage!), it's a lot trickier for a man to give extra stimulation to the head of his penis while it's inside his partner. For extra grip, he could try wearing a penis ring or a super-snug penis sleeve designed to be worn during sex (on Day Five you'll learn more about how toys can save your sex life); or the woman can make a 'V' with her index and forefinger and position it either side of her vaginal opening, so that she's gripping him between her fingers as he thrusts. She can also repetitively clench and release her pelvic muscles while he's inside her. As well as squeezing him, performed regularly these exercise will have a general strengthening and tightening effect on her vaginal walls and help make her more orgasmic too.

Extra-curricular Activity
Trading places

Looking for a really quick way to spice up your sex life? The next time you have sex, do it in a different place from wherever you did it last. Yes, a bed is usually the most comfortable place to have sex, and therefore the most likely location to help secure an orgasm – but every now and then, a change of scene is good for the soul. Doing it somewhere where there is the risk of getting caught fuels adrenalin, recreating the butterflies-in-the-stomach feeling of honeymoon-phase sex. Alternatively, simply moving to your TV-watching chair or your staircase, will force you to reposition your bodies into new angles which could throw up some sexy new sensations.

With gadgets, fingers and pelvic-floor exercises, there's a lot a woman can do to make sure she gets as much out of intercourse as her man does. More often, the thing that's *really* holding a woman back is her attitude – too many of us believe the hype, thinking, 'Well, hardly any women come through intercourse anyway, so it's OK'. Yes, it's OK to enjoy sex for sex's sake – when orgasms last only a few seconds it'd be silly to make them the soul reason for having sex. But, if you *can* enjoy an orgasm by making a little extra effort, then why not do it?

Men, on the other hand, have grown up expecting to orgasm during intercourse and may feel more frustrated by any difficulties. It's essential not to stress or obsess about that orgasm though, as the more pressure people put on themselves, the less likely they are to climax. If using rings and sleeves and finger tricks doesn't work for a man, he should try to retrain his physical responses by masturbating in a different way when he's alone – loosen that grip on a daily basis and soon his body will start to respond to lighter friction.

The Issue: You Can't Achieve Simultaneous Orgasms

It happens every time in the movies – no matter what position the couple is in – usually within forty-five seconds, and by God, they make it look good, too, don't they? No wonder we all want to do it. But they are *acting*. You could have orgasms like that too, if you were prepared to fake it – but why do it? Faking orgasms on a regular basis sabotages your sex life as you won't ever be able to address the issue as a couple when only one of you knows it exists.

Outside of Hollywood, simultaneous orgasms are rare. But they are achievable with some forward planning if you know each other's bodies well enough. Say it takes a woman around twenty minutes to reach orgasm, and it takes her partner half that time – it makes sense either to spend longer on foreplay for her or to adopt a position that's more stimulating for her and less so for him, so that he takes longer to climax.

Research shows that through masturbation, women can climax within three to five minutes, so when a man is moments away from hitting a high note, if he lets his partner know, she can flip the switch on her favourite vibe and position it at just the right spot.

However, forward planning can work against you by putting pressure on you both. Ultimately, the less stressed you feel, the more likely you are to enjoy sex – and that's the point, isn't it? Don't get too hung up on goals like simultaneous orgasms. It's OK to come separately, and from different types of sex, be it hand play, oral sex or intercourse – it can even be better that way: you get to have all the focus during your big moment, then you can enjoy watching your partner writhe in ecstasy. Surely that's just as much fun as climaxing in unison.

The Issue: He Doesn't Last Long Enough

For the record, I'm a huge fan of quickies, and if sex had to last thirty minutes every time I did it, I'd be bored senseless (and possibly a little chafed too). My point is that marathon sex sessions *can* be great fun (time and lube permitting), but five minutes of fireworks can also feel divine. Enjoying both is part of a well-rounded sex life, but if a man can only ever last a few moments then, Houston, we have a problem.

A man can learn to delay orgasm through masturbation. To do so, he should imagine a scale of one to ten, on which ten is orgasm; he should then masturbate until he reaches around a level seven, then stop and let his arousal subside back to level three or four before continuing again. By repeating this move five or six times each time he masturbates, he will start to build stamina and gain greater control over his responses.

An even simpler way to delay ejaculation is to use a condom that contains a delaying agent in the tip such as benzocaine, which mildly and temporarily desensitises the nerve endings in the head of the penis. Most reputable brands sell them, but you may need to read the labels to check which condoms have the magic ingredient, as the names don't always give the game away. For example, Durex's delaying condoms are called Performa or Performax depending on which country you're in.

During sex, a man can also withdraw just before he reaches tipping point and squeeze the head of his penis in the palm of his hand or between his fingers and thumb; he can apply firm pressure to his perineum with the tip of his forefinger; or he can tug down on his testicles. Experimenting with these moves alone during masturbation will help him to master the techniques. And masturbating before sex will also reduce the chances of coming too soon with a partner.

The Issue: She's Too Dry

Women create their own natural lubricant, secreted through the vaginal walls. Levels vary from person to person and can also depend on external factors such as alcohol consumption (if she's dehydrated, she's likely to feel drier down there, too).

Some women produce more than they need and have to dry off in order to create friction; others don't create as much as they'd like or produce it as quickly as they'd like, and so they use lube, which is a must for marathon sex sessions and anal sex, regardless.

When a woman is dry it could be her body's way of saying that she's not that turned on yet, so her partner should spend a little more time enjoying her body. If she's naturally quite dry or just dehydrated at that time, they should have fun with some lube.

One of the most interesting ways of applying lube that I've seen originated in the brothels of Bangkok. In a move called a *Bangkok Slide*, a working girl lubes up her entire body, then gets on top of her client (who may have another lubed-up working girl beneath him at the same time) and writhes all over him until he's sufficiently slippery. You could try the same move at home on a lilo or plastic sheeting, or how about a game of Twister with added lube?

In contemporary porn films, spitting on each other's genitals seems to be the most popular way to lubricate a partner, but the sight of it has me reaching for the eject button. Best check your own partner's thoughts on the matter before attempting that one!

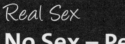

Real Sex
No Sex – Period?

I'm a porn actress and have to work regardless of whether it's that time of the month or not, but the sight of blood on set is a definite no–no, so I've discovered the way to have no-mess sex when you're on is to use natural sea sponge as a tampon. You can slide a marshmallow-sized piece of it up to the back of your vagina, and it will absorb even quite heavy flows for an hour or so. You then insert two fingers to pinch it and pull it back out. You can also buy 'soft tampons' online, which actually look exactly like marshmallows and do the same job, but I prefer the sea sponge, as it seems more absorbent.

Andrea, 26

The Issue: You've Been Faking It/You Suspect Your Partner Has Been Faking It

Not everyone realises this, but when they think they can get away with it, some men fake orgasms too. Those who use condoms will quickly discard them so the evidence is out of sight, and those who don't may claim there just wasn't very much ejaculate and hope their partner's juices or the lubricant they've been using is enough to cover their tracks.

When quizzed, men give similar reasons for faking orgasms as women do: 'I just wasn't in the mood and wanted to get it over with'; 'I'd had a little too much to drink and couldn't feel anything, but didn't want to admit that'; 'I wasn't enjoying the sex we were having, but I didn't want to hurt my partner's feelings'.

Reality check: a confident lover will accept that sometimes we just aren't in the mood, that alcohol numbs sexual sensations and that not every single sex act we ever indulge in is going to work for us; and, more importantly, that none of the above is a reflection on them. The question is: how many of us are truly confident lovers?

Everyone's confidence can get a little shaky in the bedroom, and perhaps – when incidences are isolated rather than regular occurrences – it's OK to let your lover think you've reached a climax of sorts. When it becomes a real issue is when you're living a lie, giving Oscar-worthy performances that deliberately keep your partner in the dark and prevent you from raising the issue.

If that's what you've been doing, or that's what you suspect your partner has been doing, then it's time to talk. Fakers need to put an end to their performances, but rather than saying, 'You've never made me come,' try saying, 'I'm finding it hard to come through intercourse, do you think we could try . . . [insert your own constructive suggestion here]?' If you suspect your partner of faking, rather than accusing him or her, encourage them to be open by saying, 'Is there anything I can do to make sex hotter for you?' Either way, my plan is packed with ideas to help you out of trouble.

The Issue: You Don't Feel Confident Enough to Experiment With New Positions

We can feel at our most vulnerable and exposed during sex, so experimenting with anything new can be daunting. While one glass of wine may loosen inhibitions, anything more than that will start to numb sensation, so Dutch courage isn't the best way forwards.

For women who are conscious about their bodies, lingerie is a godsend. Corsets squeeze in tummies, balcony bras create perky boobs, stockings and ruffle-bum knickers (which can be pulled to the side) help hide cellulite, and at the same time, dressing up for sex helps us to feel sexy and take on a sexually confident persona, while our lovers will be visually aroused and flattered we've made an effort for them.

If you simply can't bear to be seen in action, an alternative to lights-out sex is to introduce a blindfold. Tell your partner you want to surprise them and use a scarf, tie or stocking to cover their eyes – and hide your blushes until you've mastered a move.

Above all else, maintain a sense of humour. If you get something wrong, laugh and your partner will laugh with you – but if you curl up and die of embarrassment, they'll feel embarrassed too.

Extra-curricular Activity
X-rated copycat

If you really want to get experimental, hire an adult film and play this game. Pick a word such as 'hard' or 'cock', then settle down to watch the movie. Every time an actor says the word you've selected, you have to pause the DVD and re-enact the position on the screen at that moment.

The Issue: He's Going Soft Inside You / She's Got 'What Colour Shall We Paint the Ceiling?' Written All Over Her Face

When a session suddenly starts going off the boil, there are several quick fixes you can employ. Try whispering filthy nothings in each other's ears – generally anything that bolsters another person's ego will make them instantly feel sexier. 'You feel so good', 'I love being inside you' and 'Looking at you makes me want to explode', are the sort of one-liners that will spur a lover on.

Be more responsive; grab your lover, grind into them and don't stifle your moans – seeing and hearing you being turned on will turbo-charge their arousal.

A woman can rapidly pump her pelvic-floor muscles as though her vagina were a fist milking an udder. In facing positions a man can use his fingers to part her labia so that her clitoris is exposed and receiving maximum contact with his body. Both parties can introduce additional stimulation, such as a vibe on her clitoris or his perineum, a finger up the bottom or a mouth around a nipple.

If you think that the position you're in just isn't working, change it – but be quick to build momentum back up in the next position. Switching positions interrupts sensation and arousal – do it too often and you could go off the boil completely.

If all else fails, stop and masturbate each other or give each other oral sex for a while, then resume intercourse when you feel ready – and if you don't, who cares? Sex by hand and mouth is just as good as the genital-to-genital variety.

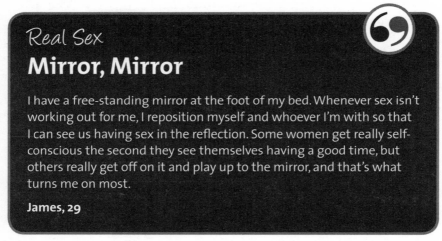

Real Sex
Mirror, Mirror

I have a free-standing mirror at the foot of my bed. Whenever sex isn't working out for me, I reposition myself and whoever I'm with so that I can see us having sex in the reflection. Some women get really self-conscious the second they see themselves having a good time, but others really get off on it and play up to the mirror, and that's what turns me on most.

James, 29

The Issue: You Can't Stay Focused During Sex

We've all been there, in the middle of a hot sex session, with our partner making all the right moves, but for some irksome reason (usually stress) we can't seem to keep our minds on the job. Random thoughts enter our heads and our internal narrators go into analytical overdrive: 'That's weird, why am I thinking about that? I should be thinking about this. Why can't I focus? What's wrong with me? What does thinking that thought even mean?' Or we find ourselves worrying about a deadline at work or a gas bill we can't afford and, before we know it, our arousal has subsided.

One way to silence your inner chatterbox is to force it to narrate the scene. Don't think about what's happening; just describe it silently to yourself in the most sexually charged terms you can think of. Force yourself into the moment by opening your eyes and watching the action.

Alternatively, dive into your own private fantasy world where deadlines and bills don't exist; turn your lover into the celebrity you most desire and your location into your dream destination.

Finally, one of the worst distractions during sex is feeling like you might need to pee, so make sure you always visit the bathroom before sex.

The Issue: He's Too Small/She's Too Big

Penis and vagina size have always been touchy subjects. It's amazing how many women who say they prefer well-endowed lovers give 'because it makes me feel small by comparison' as a reason, implying it's their ego rather than their cervix they want massaging. But it's also understandable. As women we can fret endlessly about the size of our vaginas because we have no idea what's 'normal'. We have nothing to compare ourselves against, other than our own bodies at different stages in our lives – we may be able to gauge a difference after childbirth or as we age, but we'll never be able to compare that part of ourselves to other women in the way that men can.

Perhaps it's for the best. Despite knowing (and most probably measuring up to) the average penis length of 14cm when erect, men seem to obsess about size more than women do, and an entire industry of penis enhancers and cosmetic penile surgery has been built around this paranoia, when what their lovers really need most is clitoral stimulation.

If a man falls short of the average length and his partner craves more fullness, as a general rule of thumb, the closer a woman's knees are to her chest, the deeper penetration will be, making him feel bigger inside her. So, man-on-top positions with the woman's knees pulled into her chest or hooked over her partner's shoulders, and rear-entry positions where her back is arched bringing her chest down towards her knees, will make a little go a long way.

To create a snugger fit, the best positions are those in which the woman's legs can be closed together, such as missionary or doggy-style, with both her legs positioned between her partner's.

If you're female and worried about your size, you're almost certainly worrying about nothing, especially if you haven't had children yet. If you have had children, your vaginal muscles *may* have been weakened as a result, but your midwife or doctor can examine you and prescribe a course of action. Most usually that will be pelvic-floor exercises (which you should be doing anyway as part of a healthy lifestyle), or, in extreme cases, vaginal surgery or vaginoplasty, may be the solution. There's also a range of pelvic toners on the market, ranging from electrical devices that stimulate the vaginal muscles with tiny pulses, to resistance devices that are weighted (think of a little barbell, only you hold one end inside you) or sprung (think salad tongs, inserted and then squeezed shut). You can order them all online.

The Issue: He's Too Big/She's Too Small

If a man feels too big, he should reverse the tactics above and opt for positions where the woman's legs are outstretched and open. Alternatively, any position will do, but he should stick to shallow thrusts, placing one or more cock rings around the base of his penis to create a stopper and prevent deeper thrusts. Also more lubricant should be used to prevent chafing.

For a woman who feels too small and finds intercourse painful as a result, it's statistically more likely that she's suffering from a degree of vaginismus, a common psychological condition that makes the vaginal muscles contract whenever sex is attempted.

If pain during intercourse is a regular occurrence, you must speak to your doctor who will most likely recommend psychosexual counselling (sex therapy) to help you work through any deeper issues.

The Issue: You Always Have to Initiate Intercourse

We're all creatures of habit, but it's still surprising just how little time it takes us to get into a routine way of doing things from brushing our teeth to having sex. Think about how sex usually starts with your partner, and you may soon realise that's how sex *always* starts with your partner. This can be especially frustrating for the person who always initiates intercourse.

Without recriminations, suggest a mild bondage session. If you're the initiator, ask to be tied up, so all control is passed over to your partner. They may feel like a fish out of water at first, but they may well relish the opportunity to unleash their more dominant side, while you get to play submissive for a change.

Now that you've addressed any intercourse issues you may have, and you're armed with four hot sex positions to play with and four thrusting techniques to try out, I'll leave you to enjoy the fruits of your studies! And then, on Day Five, I'll introduce you to some VIPs (very important playthings).

Day Five
Sexcessorising

Well done – you're more than halfway through *7 Days to Amazing Sex*, and if you've completed each day so far, you should be sexually fluent in hand play, oral sex and intercourse.

So, now it's time to accessorise sex with the gadgets and props that can take you all the way to sexual nirvana. An estimated one in three women owns at least one sex toy, and for today's exercises you'll need your entire collection. Don't worry if you don't have any toys, though – I'll show you how to get your hands on the perfect playthings for you. But first, let's see how much you already know about the joys of sex toys.

Exercise A
The Sex Toy Quiz – How Much Do You Really Know About Sex Toys?

Working together with your partner, spend some time considering the questions below, drawing on and sharing your own personal experience of sex aids if you have any. If not, try to guess what sex toys could bring to your bedroom party, then list your answers on a piece of paper before turning the page to see how well you've done.

Questions

1. What are the benefits of using sex aids?

2. How regularly should a person use sex toys?

3. Can a sex toy give you an STI?

Answers

1. What are the benefits of using sex aids?

Have you listed a whole bunch of signature moves that you've already mastered with your sexcessories? If so, well done – but, depending on how fluent you are in toy play, you may not have realised quite how many amazing benefits there are.

Here are just some of the ways in which modern-day sex aids can revolutionise people's sex lives:

- **They can give you more powerful orgasms.** The additional grip of a penis ring or sleeve, or the deeply penetrating sensation of vibrations reaching the parts that human touch can't, equals more intense physical responses – hold on for a super-fast orgasm!

- **They can bring variety to your solo-sex life.** Fingers can feel divine if you can climax through hand play alone. Obviously, most men can, but not all women find fingers powerful enough (which is why a lot of early female masturbation experiences involve the jet of a showerhead, long before the idea of owning a vibrator is even a consideration). Even when hand play works, it's still fun to vary your masturbation mode to keep solo sex exciting, rather than perfunctory, regardless of whether you're male or female. With so many amazing toys around now, there are hundreds of new experiences to be had. Also, playing solo with toys allows you to work on techniques that suit your body, so you can then show your lover how it's done.

- **They can satisfy fantasies.** Having a threesome is high on many people's fantasy wish lists, but the reality rarely lives up to the imagined scenario. Because people are unpredictable and emotions are involved, allowing a third person into your bed may not only turn out to be a sexual disappointment, it can also have negative implications for your relationship, leaving you or your partner feeling jealous and insecure. For some relationships, a threesome can even be fatal. However, by introducing a sex aid as the third party you can explore your fantasies safely, and at least the thrills are guaranteed. Double-penetration fantasies are easily fulfilled. Women who fantasise about the idea of sex with two men at once can ask their partner to simultaneously penetrate their free orifice with a dildo during either vaginal or anal intercourse. For the man who fantasises about having sex with two women at once, his partner can straddle his face so he can give her oral sex while she uses a lifelike masturbation sleeve on his manhood at the same time.

Some couples invest in the very expensive, but scarily lifelike Real Dolls to live out their threesome fantasies. The adult-sized silicone sex dolls, which come in both male and female models, can be customised by selecting features from height to hair colour!

Whatever your fantasy, always consider how sex aids can help you to achieve it and remember the equation: Him + Her + Any Sex Toy = The Most Physically Satisfying Threesome You'll Probably Ever Have.

Real Sex
Dolled Up

I bought my Real Doll because it was such a novelty. As a lesbian, I love the female form, and they're so beautifully crafted. Plus, I have so much fun dressing her up. My lovers have all been very impressed by her too – she's a real talking point and has taken on a character of her own. During sex, I either dress her in a strap-on, or I position a tennis ball between our genitals and roll her body up and down over mine. It's a little different to playing with a standard sex toy, but that's what makes it so much fun.

Wanda, 33

● **They can help sustain a long-distance relationship.** If you or your partner have to travel a lot for business or you live apart, sex toys can help fill the void (for want of a better expression!). You can even buy moulding kits used to make rubber replicas of a man's penis that can be fitted with a vibrator unit!

- **They can make simultaneous orgasms achievable.** If she often reaches climax before him (OK, it's rare, but not unheard of!), she can insert a vibrating butt plug into his anus, which will sit comfortably during intercourse to intensify sensation for him. If he finds he always reaches orgasm before her, he can start sessions using a vibe on her, then, when she's ready, commence intercourse in a position where he or she can keep the vibe over her clitoris. Alternatively, he can give her a three-minute 'orgasm approaching' warning during sex, to let her know it's time to switch on her vibe (with a powerful enough vibrator, a woman can reach climax in about three minutes).

- **They can help tackle penis problems.** A penis ring, worn tightly enough, can help with staying hard for longer – it works by trapping blood in an erection, while increasing sensitivity at the same time.

> *Real Sex*
> # That's Magic!
>
> I love it when my wife uses her Magic Wand during sex. At first I was a bit put out by it – it's huge! But then, when I realised it was only for external use, my ego recovered and I suggested she use it during sex, as I knew that would really get her off. What I didn't realise is what it would do to me! The vibrations are so powerful I can feel them all the way through my shaft and when she comes from holding it against her clit while I'm inside her, her muscles spasm all around me, which feels amazing.
>
> **Roger, 45**

- **They can cure anorgasmia.** Primary anorgasmia is what you're experiencing if you've never had an orgasm, and it's most likely to affect women (though in over ten years of sex research and investigation I've only ever met two women with this issue).

  Sex therapy is one way to address anorgasmia; another is to use extremely powerful vibrators to awaken sensations. In the UK, the National Health Service recommends sex aids to female patients who are unsatisfied with their sex lives; in the USA, the legendary American sexologist Betty Dodson spent a large part of her career hosting hands-on masturbation workshops for women who had difficulty achieving orgasm. Her workshops were a huge hit, with Betty leading pupils to sexual fulfilment, one orgasm at a time. Her secret weapon? The Hitachi Magic Wand – a mains-operated 'massager' and probably the most powerful sex aid in the world (see Exercise C for details).

2. How regularly should a person use sex aids?

In Days One to Four of my plan, I deliberately kept references and exercises involving toy play to a minimum. This is because it's advantageous to vary how you orgasm, alternately using fingers, tongues and genital-to-genital contact, as well as gadgets. The variety helps to keep your body tuned in to different sources of stimulation, rather than allowing it to become dependent on one particular kind. This is particularly useful for sex-on-the-go, such as that impromptu quickie in the back seat of your car, and holiday sex, when you might not have access to your treasure trove of toys.

However, some women – no matter how many alternatives they try – find they can only climax through vibration, and this is not an issue. In terms of what I call CSE (Clitoral Stimulation Effectiveness), vibes top the charts for the majority of women (tongues come second, hands third – and that leaves penises out in the cold, or, more accurately, snuggled in the warmth of a vagina, a fair distance from the clitoris).

While I'd recommend that if you are vibe-dependent, you should continue to experiment with other routes to orgasm from time to time, don't ever deny or frustrate yourselves if vibration is what you *need* to enjoy sex. Every sex act – from masturbation to intercourse – can incorporate vibe play, and, in fairness to the booming sex toy trade, you can actually buy vibes especially created for in-car use (they plug into the dashboard cigarette-lighter), and there are also several inconspicuous varieties (such as the lipstick vibe) that travel well and wouldn't raise any eyebrows during a luggage check.

3. Can a sex toy give you an STI?

The answer, unfortunately, is yes – but only if you fail to follow a few health-and-safety guidelines. Yes, I know using the words 'health' and 'safety' in the same sentence is likely to make some readers nod off, but please take a few moments to read on. The following could put you at risk:

- **Sharing toys.** Sexually transmitted infections can be spread if toys are shared without being thoroughly cleaned in between use by one person and the next. If two or more people are using the same sex toy in one session (and what a session that would be!), the toy should be dressed in a fresh condom for each new person to save having to interrupt play with the washing up.

- **Using the same toy on different parts of the body.** Condoms should also be used *and* changed between putting the same toy into other orifices after anal penetration because bacteria from the anus can be harmful in the vagina and mouth.

- **Using unhygienic toys.** When you buy a toy, it should come with cleaning instructions – these should *not* be thrown away. Cleaning a toy correctly will help it last longer and prevent the risk of genital infection from bacteria. How to clean it depends on what it's made of, and whether it has any motorised parts. Unless they're waterproof, gadgets with motors or battery packs can't be submerged in water, so a sanitised wipe should be used, whereas a glass dildo can be put through a dishwasher. Always read the instructions and regularly check toys for scratches or cracks in the surface – these are a breeding ground for bacteria, so once a toy is damaged in this way it's time to throw it away.

- **Using toys during pregnancy.** Anything that is inserted into the vagina has the potential to introduce infection to both mother and baby, so it's especially important that toys are thoroughly cleaned before being used by a pregnant woman. A doctor or midwife will advise on whether penetration (by toys or partner) is likely to cause other complications for each individual mum-to-be. For example, they may advise a woman to refrain in the early stages of pregnancy if she has a history of miscarriage or preterm delivery.

Toy envy: a modern male condition

Some men may feel a little threatened by sex toys – rather than seeing them as their tools, they're intimated by them. If that sounds like you, combat your toy envy with the following three simple steps:

1. Don't compare yourself. One issue most men have about sex toys is their size. If her toy is bigger than your penis, remember there's possibly a large battery unit at the base accounting for much of the size, and the main pleasure centre on the female body is actually the clitoris. You can't penetrate a clitoris, and most vibrators, regardless of shape or size, will be used externally. What's important is the power of the vibrations, and no man vibrates, so you can't compare yourself to something that does.

2. Own it. Rather than thinking of it as *her* vibe, think of it as yours: an extension of your sexual prowess. Get involved in the purchasing process and pay for it yourself (when it comes to romancing a long-term partner, trust me, a bunch of sex toys beats roses hands down). By literally owning the toy, you'll be able to feel responsible for the wonderful thrills it gives your lover.

3. Don't beat them – join them! Rather than harbouring negative feelings about women's use of sex toys, try to develop your own toy habit. What's good for the goose is good for the gander, right? There used to a lot of stigma regarding male sex toys, but that's no longer the case, and the male toy market is experiencing a boom. As well as the old mock vagina-style aids, which a lot of people think of as a little creepy (though my view is, if it floats your boat, keep paddling!), there are new stylised brands on the market, which don't look anything like dismembered body parts.

Developing your own toy habit will enhance your sex life, but it will also make you appreciate the limitations of sex toys. No matter how physically effective they are, they can't stir your emotions, they can't talk dirty, they can't cuddle you, or surprise you or kiss you. Once you realise this, you'll no longer feel intimidated by what they have to offer. Instead, you will see them as your sexual tools; a sex aid will assist you in creating an orgasm in the same way a power tool assists you in putting up shelves – so learn to use it!

Introducing him to your little friend

Ladies, when your sexual satisfaction is dependent on your vibe, that makes it one little friend you need your man to get along with. Some guys suffer from what I call toy envy (see p. 113) and feel threatened by either the dimensions or capabilities of sex toys. While I work with them to get over that, it's essential you help the process along. Here's how:

1. Take him shopping. Whether you buy your toys online, from a catalogue or a sex store, do it together. Opt for something small and powerful – after all it's the vibrations rather than the size that'll be of benefit to your clitoris. It might also help to pick something that isn't penis-shaped (it's a lot harder for him to compare his manhood to a vibrating butterfly or lipstick).

2. Put on a show. For your man, watching you use your toy will be like being invited to his own private sex show – regardless of his apprehensions about battery-powered gadgets, it'll be hard for him to feel anything other than *hard*, if you catch my drift. Seeing you use the toy externally will be reassuring and should put an end to the fear that you're only using toys because he's not big enough to satisfy you. If you do use the toy internally, try to eroticise that for him by saying things like, 'When I'm doing this I'm imagining you inside me'. At the same time as marrying the notion of toy play with him being turned on, you'll be feeding him info on how to use the toy on you, which will boost his confidence for when it's his turn to take the controls.

3. Spread the toy. It's odd, considering how similar the clitoris and penis are, but I've yet to meet a man who enjoys the sensation of vibrations on the head of his penis. However, the perineum and nipples are often responsive to a little massaging buzz. Try sharing the joys of your toys to see if the mutual perks can tip him towards toy appreciation.

Exercise B

Your Dream Toy – Identifying the Perfect Sex Toy For You

I've personally tested over 400 sex toys during the last 10 years and only around 50 per cent of them have hit the spot for me. Imagine how much money you could waste wading through all the toys that may not do it for you! But fear not: during this exercise you'll note down which style, size, power and noise level you prefer, and, in so doing, you'll create your Dream Toy Profile. Armed with this information, you'll know exactly what to look for (and what to avoid), regardless of whether you're shopping online, from a catalogue or in a shop, saving you both time and money. And, in the Resources section of this book (see pp. 197–201), you'll find information on where to buy good-quality toys at fair prices.

1. What's your sex toy style?

Never buy anything gold-plated or crystal-encrusted or so staggeringly high-tech that you need a degree to decipher the instructions – these mod cons add to the price rather than the pleasure. As a general rule, I've noticed that the more ostentatious a toy is, the less effective it tends to be. Instead, decide whether you'll need it to be waterproof (essential if you like a lot of fun in the tub) and then go for your favourite colours, shapes and functions.

We'll discuss different styles of sex toys in more detail a bit later, but for now think about what your sexual requirements are. For example, is your toy for solo sex or partner sex? Do you prefer external or internal stimulation, or both? Do you want a realistic-looking toy or a designer gadget? Do you need a discreet toy you can hide from your kids? Does your toy have to be waterproof?

Once you've considered your requirements, make a note of your preferred styles here:

_____

_____

_____

Vibrator volume control

Vibe volume could be a deal-breaker if you live in shared accommodation or have very thin walls. Even if you don't, a loud racket can distract some people from the orgasm in hand. In general, electric vibrators tend to be the quietest, producing a soft electric hum, while battery-powered vibes made from hard plastic make the most noise (though good-quality manufacturing can minimise this). If volume is an issue, either test toys in the shop or look for sex toy sites that give noise-level ratings.

2. Pick your power source wisely

Always buy the most powerful vibe available in the size and shape that you want. If you find that a toy is too powerful, you can always use it on a lower setting (if it's multi-speed); or, if it's for external use, you can position it to the side of, rather than directly on the area you're buzzing, or dull the vibrations by wrapping the gadget in underwear or a towel. But if you buy a vibe that's too weak, there's nothing you can do other than bin it.

- **Mains-operated electrical vibrators** are the most powerful, but of course they aren't portable. There are also fewer varieties available, and they're usually the most expensive, but you'll save money on batteries in the long run and some come with a one-year guarantee.

- **Rechargeable vibrators** come with a power dock that plugs into the mains, just like an electric toothbrush, giving you the benefit of never having to buy batteries, but they're not as powerful as mains-operated toys (and you'll still have the occasional frustration of running out of power just as you're about to orgasm). Also, while nobody has a problem leaving their toothbrush in a dock to charge, some people are a little concerned about recharging their Jack Rabbit in case their children or visitors happen to stumble across it – so it's worth considering where you'd do your recharging before buying this type of toy. Expect to find a reasonable range of designs, including several waterproof varieties, but also be prepared to pay a bit more than you would for the battery-powered equivalents.

● **Battery-powered vibrators** are the cheapest and, therefore, the most popular. They're portable, they come in so many shapes, sizes and colours that you'd be forgiven for thinking manufacturers have too much time on their hands, and several waterproof varieties are available too. If you don't like the idea of buying batteries, you can always invest in a rechargeable set. Battery-operated vibes will never be as intense as the mains-operated versions, but most are strong enough to induce orgasm. Check how many and what sort of batteries are used, and what the toy is made from – vibrations travel better through hard plastic than thick rubber.

Now, jot down which power source you think would most suit your needs:

_____

_____

Extra-curricular Activity
The sneeze test

Most shops have tester toys available, so you can gauge the noise and power levels of each vibe. To test power levels, place a toy against the tip of your nose; if the vibe makes you feel like you're going to sneeze, it's probably powerful enough to stir up an orgasm too.

3. Which material will thrill your skin?

Sex toys come in a variety of materials ranging from real-feel CyberSkin (see p. 118) to solid, shatterproof glass. What would you prefer to feel next to your skin? Here's some information on each to help you decide, listed from the most pliable to the most rigid:

● **Jelly rubber** is a soft, porous material composed of different ingredients including latex and phthalates. It's cheap and cheerful, but not very durable. A small percentage of people are allergic to latex and there has been research into the possible health risks posed by phthalates, but there is no conclusive evidence at this time to prove that phthalates in sex toys are harmful. If you're concerned, dress jelly toys in condoms before use. This will also prevent the porous material from being contaminated with hidden bacteria.

● **CyberSkin** was the first real-feel sex toy material to hit the market. Since then, new materials with names like Futurotic and UltraSkin have also become available. These materials feel *freakily* real and quickly warm to body temperature, but they're pricey, porous and difficult to clean, and need to be powdered with corn starch or flour, or tailor-made powders such as CyberSkin Renew after use (*don't* use talcum powder, which should never be put in the vagina, as it's been linked to certain kinds of cancers). As with jelly rubber, CyberSkin may also be softened with phthalates, so is best covered with a condom before use.

The eco choice

Silicone, plastics and rubber are all recyclable and some sex-toy companies now offer services where you can return old toys for recycling (some even offer a cash-voucher incentive to do so). However, metal, wood and glass toys are the best eco option: their production process is relatively non-toxic and has little environmental impact, while the toys themselves will outlast other gadgets, making them the truly green choice.

● **Silicone** is less expensive than CyberSkin, durable, hypo-allergenic, non-porous, easily cleaned and able to retain body heat. The texture can vary, but it's generally firm but flexible. This material is highly recommended.

● **Latex rubber** is quite a bit firmer than jelly and silicone toys, and it's cheaper than both, but it wears out more quickly and is porous like jelly, so can be hard to clean properly. Use a condom to protect yourself from invisible bacteria build-up and avoid it altogether if you have a latex allergy.

● **Hard plastic** transmits vibrations better than soft materials, so toys made from this could give more buzz for your buck. They're also very cheap, durable and easy to clean (but watch out for scratches on the surface that can harbour bacteria). Not everyone likes the rigidity of hard plastic, while for others, that's precisely the appeal.

● **Glass** or faux glass toys are stunning to look at and offer the rigidity that so many people love (a firm touch is particularly good for massaging his or her G-spot). Usually made from acrylic, Lucite or Pyrex, they're designed to withstand knocks and are safe to use, plus their non-porous surface is easy to clean; real glass toys can even be boiled or put through a dishwasher. The majority of glass and faux glass toys are dildos, but there is a growing number fitted with vibrator units now too. They're not cheap, but they'll last a lifetime, so long as you never chip them.

● **Wood** is a relatively new medium for sex toy manufacturers such as the aptly named NobEssence brand, and so far only dildos are available. The wood is given a chemical-free treatment to smooth the surface guaranteeing no splinters, easy cleaning and a lifetime's use. But the cost is exceptionally high.

● **Metal** toys, made from materials such as aluminum, cost-effective medical-grade stainless steel or even silver or gold for those who can afford them, are as hard as nails (obviously), they can be heated up in warm water or cooled in the fridge for added hot or

Course Notes

The cost of pleasure

When shopping for sex toys, your choice of material will affect the price. Plastic and rubber toys are among the cheapest; silicone, metal, glass and specially developed real-feel materials such as CyberSkin tend to be mid-range in price; wood and precious metals such as silver and gold are the most expensive. Consider your budget when considering your preference – for example, if you want something hard, but you're shopping on a shoestring, go for plastic rather than glass.

cold thrills and they're hygienic and sleek; but you do have to be careful in the throes of passion – a knock from one of these can really hurt (some women even keep theirs under the bed to defend against would-be burglars).

So, considering your budget and personal preferences, make a note of which materials most turn you on here:

_____

_____

Save your sex toy's life – use the right lube

Once you've decided upon the perfect material for your toy, it's time to pick an appropriate lube. Use the wrong one and you could destroy your beloved, while the right one will help to protect your investment.

- **Water-based lube** is safe to use with all sex toys and condoms, it won't stain your sheets (like silicone and oil would), and it's cheaper than silicone lube too, though it can feel a little sticky on the skin.

- **Silicone-based lube** is a more expensive option, but a little goes a long way and many people prefer the extra-slippery feel on the skin. It's also water-resistant so you can use it in the tub with waterproof toys. However, it's not compatible with silicone and CyberSkin toys as it has an erosive effect on these materials.

- **Oil-based lubes** used for sexual purposes are commonly found around the home – things like petroleum jelly or Vaseline, baby oil, hand lotion and food oils. Some lotions can upset the delicate pH balance of the genitals though, so choose carefully, opting for organic and unfragranced products or, better still, invest in a tailor-made oil-based lube. Innovative new brands such as Yes offer organic, skin-nourishing oils designed for down there. On the flip side, however, oil-based products will damage latex toys and condoms.

Now that you've created your Dream Toy Profile, you can draw up a list of potential suitors and go gadget shopping. But, before you go, I have some ideas for your existing toy collection.

Exercise C

Teach an Old Toy New Tricks – A Guide to Sex Gadgets and Their Hot Alternative Uses

Working together with your partner, gather up all the toys you have, then look them up on the list below of sexy playthings currently available on the market, along with my recommended twist for each. If there's a toy you don't have that you like the sound of, add it to your shopping list!

Girls' gadgets

Traditional 'torpedo' vibe

Like so many women, my first-ever vibe was a hard, plastic, straight up-and-down, basic torpedo-shaped model. They can be used for penetration, but most women use them externally pressing the tip on or around their clitoris, or placing them between their labia like a hotdog in a bun, allowing the vibrations to penetrate the entire vulva.

- **Twist.** Wrap a penis ring with vibrating-bullet attachment around the base of your traditional torpedo vibe to turn it into a dual-stimulation toy.

Dual-stimulation/Rabbit-style vibe

Made famous many moons ago by an episode of TV's *Sex in the City*, these double-headed vibes featuring a shaft for penetration and a smaller vibrating head for clitoral stimulation, are still as popular as ever, proving that – contrary to popular belief – women do enjoy penetration, just so long as they're getting clitoral thrills at the same time. You can even get triple-headed vibes that aim to arouse anus, vagina and clitoris all at the same time, but finding one that ergonomically matches your body shape is a real challenge.

- **Twist.** Turn your Rabbit around through 180 degrees, while keeping the shaft inside you, so that the clitoral vibe buzzes against your perineum, leaving your clitoris exposed – now invite your man to lick it!

Real Sex
Lady Luck

The one sex toy I couldn't live without is my Lady Finger. It's a plain, uncomplicated, long, thin vibe, but it really does the trick. It's perfect for rubbing over my clit, or slipping just inside my vagina – which is a really sensitive part on me – as well as rolling over my inner thighs and pubic mound. I most like to pull my knickers tight and rub the Lady Finger over the top – it's less messy and the vibrations spread out over the expanse of the fabric.

Corina, 23

G-Spot vibes and dildos

Most G-spot stimulators look like traditional vibes or dildos, but with a curved tip to help hit the spot; others have additional ripples and bulges along the shaft for increased stimulation; and there are some that are completely U-shaped (one end of the 'U' is inserted vaginally so it can place pressure on your G-spot, while the other end nestles against your clitoris – you then grip the toy and rock it back and forth to stimulate both areas). In some models the ends are also fitted with vibrating units, and there's even one U-shaped toy, called the We-Vibe, that's designed to be worn by a woman during penetrative partner sex. Who says you can't have your cake and eat it?

- **Twist.** Pop a condom on your G-spotter and try using it to locate your man's equivalent erogenous zone, his prostate, situated a few inches up inside the front rectal wall. (But if it doesn't have a U-bend, a wider base or a handle on the end, keep a tight hold of the base, so the toy can't get sucked up into his rectum.)

Real Sex
Getting Gigi with Lelo

I love the Lelo Gigi. It's a long, rechargeable vibrator made of medical-grade silicone with a very soft, flat, angled head for G-spot stimulation. It vibrates at just the right speed to get me off quickly and is very easy to keep clean and maintain. I also like to use the head to stimulate my clitoris alongside penetrative sex, especially anal and in doggy position. Guys enjoy it when I place it against my cheek during blow-jobs, too. It's a very versatile toy!

Ellen, 46

Clitoral vibes

Designed for external use only, clit-specific vibes come in a variety of shapes and guises: eggs, bullets, pebbles, butterflies and lipsticks, to name but a few. Technically, you could put them inside a vagina, but they're usually too small to make any impact.

Some plug into music players and vibrate according to the beat, some are remote-controlled, and some strap on, like the Butterfly, with elastic or plastic bands that go around the top of each thigh with another around the hips to create a harness. This helps to keep the toy positioned over the clitoris so you don't have to, leaving your hands free to roam. Other clit-stims are designed to be worn on the finger, so wherever your hands roam they take the buzz with them.

Contour vibes sit in the palm of your hand and are hugely popular with several designer varieties available like the pretty, patterned, pebble-shaped Lelo. The newest contour vibe on the market is the SaSi – as well as vibrating, a ball moves beneath its silicone skin, emulating the action of a tongue!

- **Twist.** Rather than take the bee straight to the honey (in this case, the bee being your buzzing friend, the honey your clitoris), move it around your body first. Powerful vibrations can feel particularly amazing on the nipples, abdomen and buttocks. The longer you spend building arousal and heightening the sexual tension in your body, the stronger your orgasms will be.

Real Sex
Cute Dimple

The Lelo Lily is wonderful. Shaped like a pebble with a dimple in the middle, it sits in the palm of my hand and fits perfectly against my clit – and it's much easier than manoeuvring my Rabbit into position. I like to use it during doggy-style sex. And when I'm done, it even charges up via the mains.

Katie, 27

Cone vibes

Another recent sex-toy invention, the Cone, was created by a guy I met at an Erotic Awards ceremony (the Cone won). He explained that he'd actually been trying to invent a BDSM (see p. 80) seating device for sexually submissive women who get off on pain, but rather than take his guinea pigs to their pain/pleasure limits, the device only gave them pleasure, and so, a new mainstream sex toy was born. It's an acquired taste: you sit on it, and while its vibrations travel through your entire vulva, it stretches the vaginal opening – a sensation some women love, but personally, I find a little uncomfortable.

- **Twist.** Place the Cone on a chair and while you lower yourself up and down as far as you can go, have your man kneel between your legs and lick you to orgasm.

Electric massagers

It's impossible to say 'electric massager' without thinking of the Hitachi Magic Wand, the most popular of the hand-held plug-in devices used in the bedroom – though it has to be said, this is genuinely good for massage too. My husband uses it on his legs to combat running injuries and my mother-in-law found it helped with her sciatica; it's also great for facial massages and helps tone the chin and jowls. The turbo-charged vibrations that make it so effective for all forms of massage are also the reason it's become famous as a masturbation tool for women. If you've never had an orgasm, or find it very difficult to orgasm even when masturbating with standard vibes, this is the toy for you. However, the very thing that makes this gadget so marvellous may also be its downfall, because by allowing your body to become accustomed to such intense vibrations, you may condition your genitals to become unresponsive to lesser forms of stimulation. If you find you develop a Hitachi habit, whereby other forms of stimulation cease to work for you when once they did, it's time for rehabilitation! Begin by using the lower setting on the Wand, then switch to a less powerful battery-operated toy, and finally start to alternate between vibe and fingers. It's for your own good!

- **Twist.** Use the Wand to massage your man's perineum. Nestle the head just behind his testicles, and push it firmly up against his body using your weaker hand. While the vibrations power through his flesh, reaching his internal G-spot or prostate, use your dominant hand to masturbate him at the same time. He'll love it.

Real Sex
Electric Dreams

The Hitachi Magic Wand really upped the stakes in my solo-sex life. I usually find it really hard to come, but the wand can go on for ever, as it doesn't rely on batteries. It's quite expensive, but it does come highly recommended by sex therapists. If I hold it against my clitoris for too long, even on the slowest setting (there are two different speeds), it can get desensitised. The trick is to apply plenty of lube and use it on the whole genital area and on your body as well.

Bea, 30

Ben Wa/duotone balls

There's a lot of confusion over the naming of these little balls. Traditionally, Ben Wa balls (also known as Geisha balls) are a pair of loose, metal, marble-sized balls that are either solid or hollow with a weighted ball inside. They're inserted into the vagina and held in place by the muscles for use as a form of pelvic workout and/or a very subtle pleasure-giver. Heavier balls are better for workouts (you have to grip harder to stop them falling out), while weighted balls create more internal movement for pleasure – but you have to be extremely sensitive to feel anything at all when using these gadgets alone. They can, however, be worn during penetrative sex to provide interesting new sensations for you and your partner. When you're finished with them you can squeeze them out with your muscles, hook them out with your fingers or, if they're connected by string, you simply pull the loop at the end, just like a tampon (but beware of cheap, uncovered, absorbent cords that can harbour all manner of germs).

The larger varieties, which are around the size of golf balls, are most commonly known as duotone balls, but are also sometimes referred to as Ben Wa balls, or by brand names such as Smartballs. Some sets even have three or four balls, all attached by cord (with more than two balls, you might want to leave one outside your body to provide some external stimulation as you move around). The balls are generally hollow, made of hard plastic and coated in soft materials such as silicone, which also covers the connecting cord for hygiene reasons; weighted balls inside the spheres or attached vibrating units provide stimulation for the wearer.

- **Twist.** Insert balls inside the vagina, then use a powerful vibrator to set them in motion.

Boy's Toys

Penis rings

Individual rings are either worn around the base of the penis or around the base of the penis and testicles together, while dual penis rings feature individual hoops for each. They come in many different materials including rubber, leather, silicone and metal (though I would strongly advise novices against using solid metal rings as they can get stuck). Some have 'tickle' tassels and/or clitoral vibrators attached for the benefit of female partners.

Rings allow blood into the penis but restrict the flow out, trapping blood in an erection, keeping it harder for longer and increasing sensation for some wearers. However, they should never be worn for more than thirty minutes at a time, as too much blood pressure can damage delicate penile tissue. Also, always keep a tube of lube handy – it's useful for helping rings to slip off.

- **Twist.** When using a vibrating ring, position the vibrating unit (designed to buzz against her clitoris) under your testicles, so your perineum feels the vibrations instead. Alternatively, wrap the rubber band twice or three times around a finger to make an improvised finger vibe.

Real Sex

Great Balls of Desire

My girlfriend gave me an Adam and Eve CyberSkin Double Pleasure Masturbator – it's a masturbation sleeve with two sets of balls inside, and it has to be one of the best inventions ever! It provides good grip and, when lubricated, it's really easy to use. The small balls inside stimulate all the right areas, and it's great because I can use it alone for self-pleasure or with my partner, who provides the added luxury of putting her tongue on the tip of it, so she can lick the head of my penis with every thrust. Pure bliss.

Freddie, 39

Masturbation sleeves

Made from materials such as jelly rubber or silicone, these soft tubes are designed for penetration. Some are fitted with vibrating units, others have rippled internal surfaces or small beads embedded within the material for extra stimulation and some are shaped to look like a mouth, vagina or bottom (with inner dimensions varying accordingly).

Either a man or his lover can use a lubed sleeve to enhance masturbation for him and they feel sensational, but using sleeves – particularly those that resemble body parts – does have a sleazy image. This is unfair, considering the number of imitation penises women use to get off, but that may all be about to change with amazing new brands on the market that look more like designer toiletries – and, in the case of the much lauded Tenga Flip, iPod docks.

- **Twist.** To give sleeves a more sensual and real (vagina) feel, heat lube to body temperature by placing the unopened bottle in a bowl of hot water before squirting some into the sleeve.

Real Sex
Flipping Brilliant!

I love the Tenga Flip Hole, because: a) unlike a lot of blokes' toys it actually works; b) it recognises that the more you attempt to recreate in a toy the look and feel of a vagina, the less it looks and feels like one; and c) it neither feels like sex nor bog-standard masturbation – it's a new and extremely interesting third way of having sex. Also, unlike even the best sleeves, this one's really easy to clean, as the tube's encased in plastic which flips open – hence the name – and you can run it under a hot tap before use for extra warmth and juiciness.

Al, 40

Penis extenders

Also known as 'French ticklers', extenders look like masturbation sleeves with a head on the end and the ripples are usually on the outside for her pleasure, rather than on the inside for his. Some are also fitted with a vibrator at the base. They're worn over the penis to increase width and/or girth, but there's not much in it for the male wearer unless he suffers from premature ejaculation, as this device considerably reduces sensation for him.

- **Twist.** Place an extender on her favourite toy to bulk up its dimensions. (Note: for vaginal penetration only – extenders can very easily get lost in anal cavities).

Prostate massagers

Designed to massage the male G-spot, some are U-shaped, with one end entering the anus, the other pressing against his perineum (the perineum end may also be fitted with a bullet vibrator). Others are, loosely speaking, T-shaped like the Aneros (one of the best on the market). Made from rigid plastic, one end goes in the bottom, another then nestles against his perineum and the third end is a handle used for insertion and extraction only; this is a battery-free, hands-free device moved by him clenching and releasing his anal muscles.

- **Twist.** While he stimulates his own G-spot with a tailor-made massager, she can give him oral sex – an experience guaranteed to go straight into his Top 10 Sex Encounters of All Time.

His 'n' Hers Thrillers

Butt plugs

Available in a variety of materials, from jelly rubber to medical-grade steel, butt plugs are specially shaped anal fillers. They're usually pointed at the tip to facilitate easier entry, wider in the middle to provide that feeling of fullness, narrow at the neck to help keep them in place and flared at the base to prevent them from getting involuntarily 'sucked up' by the rectal muscles. In addition, some have design features, such as ponytails protruding from the flared end. Lubricant is essential for insertion.

Some vibrate, others just sit there in the anal cavity while wearers indulge in whatever additional sex acts they enjoy, from masturbation to oral or vaginal sex. Orgasm is generally intensified as a result.

- **Twist.** Turbo charge a standard butt plug by pushing the head of a powerful vibrator against the flared base to send vibrations up through the plug and into the rectum.

Anal beads

Also sometimes known as Thai beads, these toys comprise a line of several beads in varying sizes and are usually made of plastic, rubber or silicone. Avoid beads connected by bare string for hygienic reasons; instead, choose beads connected by cord which is coated in rubber or silicone, and therefore easier to clean.

The beads are lubricated, then inserted, one by one, into the bottom. They are then slowly pulled back out again (by either the wearer or their partner), usually just before or at the point of orgasm. Some also have a vibrating unit at the end, which is left outside the anus.

- **Twist.** Making sure your anal beads are thoroughly sterilised – or, to be super safe, before you've used them anally for the first time – try this clitoral-stimulation trick: holding each end, run the balls up and down between well-lubricated labia so the balls repeatedly bump over the clitoris.

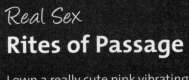

Real Sex
Rites of Passage

I own a really cute pink vibrating butt plug, which I sometimes wear during sex. Having penetration going on in the back passage makes the penetration going on in the front feel much tighter, plus the vibrations travel through the walls of my bottom into my vagina, so my husband benefits too.

Christina, 49

Dildos

Dildos are used vaginally and anally and come in a wide range of materials, from soft rubber to solid, shatterproof glass. These non-vibrating toys are either free-standing, fitted with a suction cup at the base (so they can be stuck to surfaces such as chair seats or shower cubicle walls and backed on to) or specially designed to be attached to strap-on harnesses. Sales of strap-on dildo and harness sets to straight couples (where the male enjoys anal penetration) have increased notably in recent years as the stigma attached to straight men enjoying anal sex has decreased.

There are even strap-on sets where the dildo is attached to the harness over the chin for men to wear while giving their partner oral sex (assuming their partners can stop laughing long enough to enjoy an orgasm).

Dildos provide a feeling of fullness and internal stimulation for the person being penetrated, while some harnesses are fitted with an internal dildo and/or clitorial stimulator for female wearers.

- **Twist.** Play with chill thrills by placing your dildo in a fridge before use.

Condoms

Condoms are made from either latex or polyurethane (good for those with latex allergies), and while they're not often seen in sex toy listings, I'm on a one-woman crusade to have them recognised as such. Yes, they can save your life and protect you from nasty STIs and unwanted pregnancies, but the new condoms on the block can also help to improve your sex life. Try flavoured condoms to make safe oral sex taste so much sweeter, or use condoms with added stimulation lubes – some contain heating agents to make sex extra hot, while others contain mint for added tingles.

- **Twist.** Customise condoms and enhance sensation for the wearer by adding a few drops of your own favourite lube inside the teat before application.

Real Sex
Strapping Lass

After quite a few drinks, my boyfriend admitted to me that he masturbated anally. I was quite shocked at first, as we hadn't even gone as far as me sticking a finger up his bum. I'm a little squeamish about doing that, to be honest, but I figured he'd brought it up because it was something he wanted me to be involved in. I had the idea to buy a strap-on, as I was more comfortable penetrating him with something other than my finger. The gender role-reversal really appealed to me too. The first time we tried it, I didn't do a good job; I was too rough and caused him more pain than pleasure. I think I got a little carried away on a power trip having that thing between my legs! But the second time I was slower, gentler and used way more lube and it was great for both of us. The inside of the harness rubbed against my clit, and my boyfriend masturbated as I entered him doggy-style. Being the thruster for a change also made me really appreciate how much physical effort men make and I'd definitely recommend it to other couples.

Carla, 26

After Day Five of *7 Days to Amazing Sex* you should be buzzing in more ways than one! You'll have mastered the toys of the trade and learnt how to deliver electric orgasms. But now it's time to prepare yourself for Day Six when you'll be learning how to use the most exciting sex toy you'll ever play with: your brain.

Day Six

Erotica, Role Play and Communication

Over the last five days, you've learnt how to have mind-blowing sex in a variety of ways; you've uncovered erogenous zones, tried exciting new techniques and mastered the art of toy play. But make no mistake: this will be nothing more than a quick fix for your love life if you do not now learn how to *speak* sex. And it's an awkward language for many.

A lot of us have been brought up to believe it's 'rude' to talk about sex and, as a result, our sexual vocabularies are painfully limited – but, just like any foreign language, it can be learnt, and it can also be very sexy! Once you've completed *7 Days to Amazing Sex*, this language will be key to its continuing success. Why? Because when you're able to engage in open and fluid sex dialogue, you can address any sexual problems that arise in future, you'll feel confident enough to suggest new moves (no matter how kinky you think they are) and you'll be able to articulate your desires and dislikes without offending your partner.

But how many times have you read that communication is the key to good sex? We've *all* heard it before, and on receiving this hackneyed given, most people roll their eyes and lose interest. If that's you, stop right there. My plan is different from any other sex guide you've ever read and my method for bringing communication into the bedroom is going to turn you on, rather than switch you off.

So, proceed with an open mind and prepare to discover the joys of the other kind of oral sex.

Exercise A

Story Time – A Crash Course in Talking Dirty

In 2004, I launched a glossy lifestyle magazine for women in the UK called *Scarlet*. I wanted the magazine to be as frank and forthright as the existing mainstream men's magazines of the time, catering to female sexuality in the same way that lads' mags had been doing for the boys for years.

The trouble was, that while magazines like *Maxim* and *FHM* could pose female models in convincing and sexy states of arousal – swollen, naked breasts, open legs, arched backs and orgasmic facial expressions – it was very difficult to portray arousal in male models because it was, and remains, illegal to show an erection in a mainstream British magazine. And without one, men simply don't look very turned on.

We still showed off men's topless bodies, but – as glorious as the male torso is – this didn't have quite the same impact as seeing a man fully engorged. So, unable to change censorship laws, *Scarlet* instead offered an alternative form of titillation to its readers: erotic fiction.

It was a bigger success than we could ever have hoped for. Thousands of readers wrote in to tell us that our erotic fiction supplement, called *Cliterature*, had changed their sex lives. And, what's more, their boyfriends and husbands started writing to us too, saying how much they'd enjoyed reading the stories with their partners.

It very quickly became clear that erotic fiction, as well as being a lot

Course Notes

Lead them on

As your partner's reading to you, offer encouragement: stroke their leg or their hair (nothing more – you're trying to encourage, rather than distract), and offer the occasional, 'Wow, that sounds sexy'. It's OK to giggle if they do, but after you've had a laugh, get back into arousal mode and put yourself into the story.

of fun, was a tool that could revolutionise couples' sex lives, and in this exercise I'm going to show you how.

The following extracts are from a selection of my favourite *Cliterature* capers, cherry-picked and edited by me for you to enjoy. But I don't just want you to read them. For this exercise, I want you to ask your partner to choose the story theme that most appeals to them from the Contents list below, then read that story out loud to them.

If you've never 'talked dirty' before, this is a great way to start. The pressure's off, as you don't have to think of what to say, only how you say it. Read slowly and softly – lowering your volume and slightly deepening your tone will add instant sex appeal to your voice.

Contents

She Lets Him Watch (p. 136)
Theme: female masturbation in a game of 'show and tell'

The Curtain Twitchers (p. 138)
Theme: male masturbation in the great outdoors

A Husband and Wife Share a Toilet Break (p. 140)
Theme: vanilla sex – as in the ice cream: the most basic flavour and the most popular, aka straight penetrative sex

A Lover Offers Herself for Dessert (p. 142)
Theme: oral sex for her with some food play thrown in

Things to Do Before You Die (p. 143)
Theme: oral sex for him at the Mile-high Club

The Power of Three (p. 146)
Theme: threesomes – the MMF (two males, one female) variety in this case

The Night Nina and Olivia Met (p. 148)
Theme: lesbian sex, guest-starring a big, black strap-on

Two Men and a Tub (p. 149)
Theme: homeoerotica – erotica featuring homosexuality, which, in recent years, has become hugely popular with heterosexual women; and, yes, straight men can enjoy it too, erotica being designed to stimulate fantasies, many of which you'll never need (or want) to act upon

Mixing Business and Pleasure (p. 151)
Theme: BDSM – extreme sex play in the office

She Lets Him Watch

I still remember the first woman who brought herself to orgasm in front of me. We didn't know it at the time, but this – the two of us, naked on my bed – would become a habit. But at this moment, it was all fresh, and I shivered with excitement at the sight of her reclining on a large pillow against the wall. 'Will you touch yourself for me?' I asked.

She pinched her own nipples, fondling and teasing her breasts. 'Are you just going to watch?' she asked, looking at my cock sticking out at her in the most provocative way. 'If I'm going to give you a show, you need to give me one as well.'

'Sure . . . ' I began.

I took up position at the foot of the bed, facing her, our feet touching. She lifted one knee, resting it against the wall on one side of the bed, giving me the best look I had ever had at her pussy. Her inner labia were compact, only visible peeking out from between the thick outer lips when aroused. Later, they would glisten, their colour a bright pink between the light brown curls of her pubes. This evening, I recall in photographic detail, it had been a while since she'd done any downstairs styling, and she lovingly brushed the hair aside with her fingers, teasing herself and me before running the tip of one finger along her slit. I could smell her from across the bed, her own olfactory signature of arousal. I still miss that scent sometimes.

For what seemed like a long, long time her index finger traced the edges of her sex until she dipped it inside, quickly, just enough to coat it with lubrication up to the first knuckle. She circled the wet tip around her clit, not touching, just teasing.

I think she may have forgotten I was there, that she was putting on a show. Her eyes closed, and, a hand kneading one of her breasts, she fell into a rhythm of dip–circle, dip–circle, her finger entering progressively deeper with each repetition, then more fingers joined in. The pace intensified. Her left hand became involved. She stuck two fingers into her mouth for licking, then she shoved them deep inside herself. Meanwhile, the fingers of her right hand, now dripping wet, concentrated on her clitoral hood, rubbing harder, faster, occasionally giving a soft, wet slap on top of the clit.

Eyes still closed. 'How . . . do . . . I look?' she purred.

'Gorgeous,' I croaked, my throat dry with excitement. I wasn't watching her fingers or her glistening sex any more – I was staring at her face.

Too shy to talk?

If you simply can't bring yourself to talk sex, not even to read an erotic story, I need you to take a leap of faith with me and trust me when I tell you the first words are always the hardest – after that, you'll be surprised at how easy it gets. Here are a few tricks you can try to help overcome that first hurdle:

- If you've never been much of a talker in the bedroom, one way to lift the self-imposed silence is to start talking during solo masturbation sessions. You'll feel silly at first, but not as self-conscious as you would if a lover was present in the room. After a while, as your arousal levels increase, your self-consciousness will take a back seat. If you're lost for words, talk about how you feel, describe exactly what you're doing or narrate a sexual fantasy out loud. Notice which taboo words have a direct impact on your arousal – do certain words turn you on, while others turn you off? Make a mental note of this information, as it will be invaluable to the lover who wants to talk dirty to you.

- Read an erotic story, recount the best sex you've ever had with your partner or a sexual scenario you'd like to try with them over the phone. This saves them seeing your blushes and you can masturbate while you do so to help get you in the right mindset (plus, masturbating does wonders for effecting a sexy, breathy voice). This can also be a lot of fun if your partner happens to be in their workplace at the time, unable to respond and faced with the task of having to hide their arousal from colleagues.

- While talking dirty when your partner is present, blindfold them to help them fully absorb themselves in the tale you're telling, and/or ask them to masturbate as you talk. Their averted gaze will make you feel less self-conscious, and having them pleasure themselves will take some of the attention away from you.

'I'm going to fuck you later,' she mumbled, without opening her eyes. Then she came. For a moment I felt like she wasn't there – like she had folded into herself. Her limbs curled, she rolled on her side hiding her face in my pillow and screamed. No modest little whimper for her. This was a full-throated wail from the belly on up, and, when she was done, she lay very still, cupping herself with both hands as if protecting her oversensitive clit from the world and from me. I kissed her arm, then her neck, not knowing that right at this moment an addiction was being born.

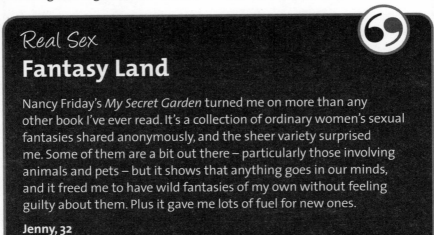

Real Sex
Fantasy Land

Nancy Friday's *My Secret Garden* turned me on more than any other book I've ever read. It's a collection of ordinary women's sexual fantasies shared anonymously, and the sheer variety surprised me. Some of them are a bit out there – particularly those involving animals and pets – but it shows that anything goes in our minds, and it freed me to have wild fantasies of my own without feeling guilty about them. Plus it gave me lots of fuel for new ones.

Jenny, 32

The Curtain Twitchers

'You've got to see this.' I led Claire to the kitchen window that overlooked our neighbour's back lawn. After watching the spectacle in Mrs Neil's garden a couple of times on my own, I'd decided it was only polite to share the view with my live-in lover. As a fellow bisexual, I knew she'd appreciate the view.

'Who is he?' she whispered.

'Mrs Neil hired him a couple of months ago. I don't know his name.' I grabbed Claire's arm and we gave a collective gasp of appreciation as the man slipped his T-shirt over his head, exposing a smooth chest with nipples the colour of ripe peaches.

'Maybe we should get a gardener too,' Claire whispered. The fact that we didn't have a garden seemed irrelevant as we watched him wipe down his hot, sweaty body with the discarded T-shirt, the strokes like caresses.

Our eyes followed the movement of his hand across his broad chest, over his hard stomach, and soon it became apparent that Mrs Neil's gardener was well on his way to an erection that his tightly fitted shorts could barely contain. We both craned our necks and squinted harder.

'He'll see us! Get back,' I hissed. As I pushed Claire behind the edge of the curtain, my hand brushed the soft curve of her breast.

She had just got out of the shower, and was draped in the red silk robe that I always wanted to stroke. The fabric clung damply to her curves. She smelled clean and citrusy, and I could just make out a hint of her own earthy musk, which made the muscles of my vulva clench and tingle.

I couldn't keep from wondering whether she'd pleasure herself over the sight of the gardener next door, and that thought made me almost as wet as watching him myself.

As we continued to spy on him, he checked the high wooden gate to make sure it was securely locked, then gave the rest of the garden a walkabout before stretching out on the wide stone bench near the fish pond. When he'd made himself comfortable and was no longer looking our way, we moved back from behind the curtain for a better view.

Like in a dream he slid his hand under the waistband of his shorts and shifted until he was satisfied with the grip. 'Come on,' Claire urged, 'unwrap it. Let's see some cock.'

It was almost as though he'd heard her. As we watched, he lifted his hips and slipped his shorts down over the rounded cheeks of his butt. His cock was heavy and thick, and we had a clear view of his weighty balls, which he cupped and stroked in their nest of dark curls. His other hand encircled his rapidly engorging penis, stroking loosely from base to tip, pausing occasionally to caress the head, which seemed to be deepening in colour with growing arousal, becoming several shades darker than his taut nipples.

With her arm draped around my shoulder, Claire's robe gaped just enough to give me a luscious glimpse of one of her breasts. I squirmed around, the intriguing heaviness of arousal spreading rapidly between my legs.

Now my attention was divided between the man stroking himself in the garden and Claire, whose other hand had disappeared beneath her robe, sweeping back and forth across her own sex.

'What do you think would happen if we just went next door and joined him, just slipped right on to his cock and had a ride?' she asked as her rocking quickened. It was too much to resist. I parted my legs and – standing right there at the window – grabbed my pussy, matching her pace.

Soon the gardener was bucking hard against his own stroking palm and Claire turned her attentions to me, spreading me with fingers already soaked by her own wetness. I still couldn't take my eyes off the man next door; his cock was now darkly engorged, so heavy and full that the weight of it seemed to be making the muscles in his pumping forearm bulge from the effort. As his strokes had become faster, so did Claire's and I felt the tightness of desire grip me. When the glistening line of come shot from him like a fountain, I could no longer hold back the explosion of my own orgasm. Wave after wave of pleasure flowed through me, and I knew the gardener was one man I'd never want to meet, but would never forget.

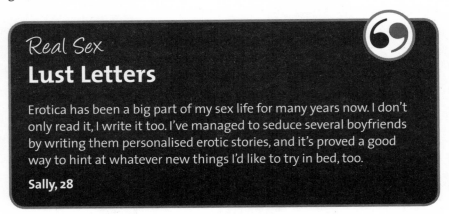

Real Sex
Lust Letters

Erotica has been a big part of my sex life for many years now. I don't only read it, I write it too. I've managed to seduce several boyfriends by writing them personalised erotic stories, and it's proved a good way to hint at whatever new things I'd like to try in bed, too.

Sally, 28

A Husband and Wife Share a Toilet Break

'Shhh,' he whispered, pulling me around so I was facing him. 'Just be quiet for once.' Then he put his hand on the back of my neck and pulled my face in close to his, gently licking just between my lips – a move he knew would make me wet.

I opened my mouth to him, but he moved away, finger on lips, motioning silence, then led me into one of the toilet stalls, manoeuvring me so my back was against the door and my wrists were pinned above my head in one of his hands.

As he pushed hard against me I could feel the hot pressure of his erect cock against my thigh and I was desperate to free it from his jeans, but I couldn't move. He yanked my dress up around my waist, tongue diving deeply into my mouth, all the while. I moaned quietly, struggling to spread my legs so he could reach my wet pussy, swollen now and longing for his fingers, his tongue, his cock . . . Then I felt his hand slip beneath my knickers, fingertips gently tracing the lines of my dripping labia. I shuddered, grinding myself against him, desperate for more friction.

When a woman came in to use the toilets we were occupying at our local restaurant, I was audibly groaning, so he whipped his hand out of my pants and planted it firmly over my mouth. I could smell my own arousal on his hand and my hips bucked into him of their own accord.

We stood like that for what seemed like for ever, eye to eye with my heat growing every second, until we heard the flush and the swing of the door that meant we were alone again. After that, there was no time to waste. Tangling his fingers in my soaking pants, he peeled them down my thighs and I opened myself to his eyes and hands. Burning energy coursed through me as he teased my clit, then he looked at me with a question in his eyes. I nodded, barely moving, pinned against the door now by the force of my own desire.

My eyes fastened on his crotch as he unbuttoned his jeans and revealed his beautifully erect cock. The feeling of his hardness rubbing against my soaking pussy was too much to bear; I braced myself against the wall and lifted my hips to him as he slowly – oh so slowly – slid inside me. As his warmth filled me I moaned again, biting my lip in a vain attempt to muffle the sound. My eyes were locked on to his as I took in all of him, gasping at the sweet pain of it.

And there we were, pressed together, the curve of his groin pushing hard against my tender clit as he gently moved inside me; with each rock of his hips I got closer, panting for breath and gritting my teeth, feeling something delicious build inside me. His nails dug into the soft flesh of my bottom, and I knew I was close. Pumping my body against his, my orgasm soaked out from my hot, tight pussy as I clenched myself around him one final time and felt his wetness rush inside me. He collapsed against me, shaking, spent; the salty sweat of his brow mingling with my own.

Real Sex
Sweet Sugar Daddy

My favourite erotic book is called *Daddy's Girl* by Stella Black. I've read it at least three times and could read it a dozen more and not get bored. It's clever, and funny, and it makes me feel incredibly horny. It's the real-life story of a woman who, in her mid-twenties, had a seven-year affair with a man in his mid-forties. He was rich and had time on his hands to come up with diverse sexual scenarios. Although I'm neither into BDSM or father/daughter role-playing, I tuned into the domination and control aspects of their relationship. It revealed aspects of my own character that I haven't yet fully explored and that touched a nerve.

Suzanne, 45

When it was finished we pulled apart slowly, almost embarrassed. As good as it was with us, it had never been like this. I kept my eyes down, as I pulled my pants up and fixed my dress. Then I pushed the door open and made my way to the sink. He followed me, stood behind me for a second, then grabbed my hand and squeezed it. I returned the pressure and met his gaze in the mirror. He looked wild, dishevelled, gorgeous. He winked at me in the mirror as he bent to kiss my shoulder, then he dropped my hand and left as quietly as he'd come in.

A Lover Offers Herself for Dessert

I lay on the kitchen table as directed, legs bare and spread wide, my skirt pushed up around my waist, shirt open, exposing my breasts. My nipples were hard points of expectation, rising and falling as I breathed heavily.

'Deborah,' he said and leant over to kiss me. I always think you know what a new lover will be like from their kiss and I felt my clit bristle with envy as Jack teased my mouth with his own. He sucked and nibbled my lips, then swirled his tongue around mine. It felt good, no clashing of teeth, not too much pressure, just right. So I shamelessly pushed his shoulders down, inviting him to taste between my legs.

The pointed tip of his tongue gently sliced through my labia causing my back to arch and my breasts to swell. I grabbed his hair, pulling his face into my wanton flesh; I needed him to eat me. He shook his head, 'Such a greedy girl,' then brought his lips back to my mouth. He tasted of me: sweet and musky.

Then, smiling, he walked over to his fridge and reached in for something I couldn't at first see . . . it was a carton of something . . . a carton of Madagascan vanilla cream.

He drizzled a cool, wet trail over my curves, authoritatively kneading my breasts, his thumbs flicking across my nipples with each stroke. 'It's delicious,' he commented and stooped to lick my nipples clean. I felt an invisible thread from each one tugging my sex from deep inside. Desperate for his touch, I clamped my legs together trying to squeeze my own aching clit.

Ripples of goose bumps and anticipation spread across my skin as he began to pour the cream again, this time in a line down my stomach leading towards my . . .

'Legs apart,' he ordered. Obediently, I opened them and gasped with excruciating delight as the cream landed on my clit. Each tiny splash sent jolts through my body and I strained to spread my legs wider, then wider still as I felt the cool liquid trickle all the way down to the crevice of my buttocks.

My hand reached down to my craving clitoris, but Jack grabbed it and placed it above my head. 'That's what my tongue's for,' he said, smiling – and then I felt it.

Heat enveloped me, blood engorged me and the world disappeared as he sucked my clit into his warm, wet mouth. His tongue flickered against me, beating in time to the spasms in my groin. With each stroke, an intense orgasm grew inside me, threatening to burst at any moment. Then he stopped.

I shook with urgency and begged him, 'Please – fuck me with your tongue, Jack. Eat me, eat me, please,' I implored. And then there was that smile of his again. But not for long. As his face disappeared once more, buried in my wetness, I flung my head back and howled. I'd never been licked so hard, so frantically, so greedily. And then, as he pumped three fingers inside of me, curling them up to push against the fleshy nub of my engorged G-spot, the banks of my orgasm finally burst.

Limp in his hands, with the world coming back into focus, a satisfied sigh escaped my lips and the aroma of vanilla was lodged in my memory for ever.

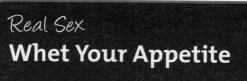

Real Sex
Whet Your Appetite

Tasting Her, edited by Rachel Kramer Bussel, is an amazing collection of oral-sex stories. Too many women worry about how they smell or taste down there – this book helps you get over that. It's also full of inspiring scenarios, like the one where a woman has a glass of wine balanced on her tummy that she isn't allowed to spill while her boyfriend goes down on her – so hot!

Sarah, 29

Things to Do Before You Die

Frankly, I'd gone on holiday to get laid. Unfortunately though, I must have picked the wrong season for sex. Then, at passport control on the way home,

I spotted them: two super-cute guys, one with a shaved head and broad shoulders, the other with fair hair and a cheeky face. They both looked like good fun.

I remarked on their matching T-shirts (they were returning early from a stag do and this was bachelor party uniform, apparently), and so we got chatting. The blond was called David; the other was called Neil. After they got their seat allocations, they hung around while I got mine, and, as we were all together in a row of three, they suggested sharing a few drinks at the bar before take-off. It was as if they'd read my mind, and, all of a sudden, a ten-hour return journey from Vegas didn't seem like such a drag.

The drinks flowed, and I began to fantasise about being the piggy in the middle on the plane, both their hands under my blanket, fighting to get their fingers inside me. When we got round to asking each other what we did for a living, I lied and said I was lap dancer (I work in insurance), and the conversation quickly took a turn for the better.

'Don't you get freaked out by men ogling at you all the time?' Neil asked.

'No,' I replied. 'I love the idea of turning guys on – there's nothing hotter than an aroused man.' My encouragement and the Dutch courage provided by the alcohol spurred them on, and by the time we boarded I'd been asked who, out of David and Neil, I found most sexy.

'I'll have to think about that for a while,' I said, taking the seat between them. 'Maybe I can tell you after a few hours, when I've gotten to know you both a bit better ...'

The next few hours were excruciating. I could feel every inch of my swollen pussy as Neil's leg purposely rested against mine on one side, while to the left, David's hand constantly brushed my own. It was like the world's most innocent threesome. Then, once the lights were out and the other passengers were focusing on getting some sleep, David also drifted off and Neil and I continued whispering conspiratorially.

'When the rest of the stags get back, there's no way they'll believe I was sat in the Mile-high seats with a lap dancer,' said Neil.

'What are Mile-high seats?' I asked.

'The ones right next to the loos,' he said. 'Makes it easier to slip in there and do ... you know, without getting caught.'

You're actually on the worst seats in the plane, precisely because they're right next to the toilets and you're sitting with an insurance clerk, I thought, but I preferred Neil's take on things, and so left him with the fantasy.

'Are you a Mile-high member, then?' I asked.

'No, but it's on my list of things to do before I die,' he said.

'Well,' I said, 'you never know when your plane's gonna crash . . . ' and I flashed my eyes in the direction of the cubicle. 'Shall I follow you in there in a sec?'

Neil was gone in a flash and I quickly joined him. His jeans were already undone and a proud, hard member greeted me. I dropped to my knees and inhaled him. Divine. Gripping the base, I dribbled my hot saliva over the head of his cock and used the wetness to stroke my hand up and down his shaft. The muscles in his thighs bulged and his hips rocked back and forth, begging me to pick up pace. Teasing him a moment longer, I circled my tongue around the ridge before sucking the head between my lips. Oh, how I love that taste: salt and musk and man. He filled my mouth and gripped my hair as my tongue rode up and down his length followed by my hand. I felt his veins pumping and knew it would be over soon. I didn't want it to end, but as I tried to slow down he thrust into me, needy and urgent, and already too close to change course. Looking up, I saw his gorgeous face contort in pleasure as warmth flooded my throat. Neil had come – a lot.

Returning to my seat a few moments after Neil, I saw that David was awake and not looking best pleased. 'You OK?' I asked later when Neil had fallen into a post-coital slumber.

'Ignore me,' said David. 'I'm probably just jealous.'

'There's no need to be,' I offered. And soon, I was back in the cubicle, this time having my needs met by David's skilful tongue and fingers as I stood back to the wall with one foot perched on the toilet seat, knickers ripped to the side, climaxing around his hand.

Real Sex
Bowled Over

Erotic fiction isn't just a turn-on – it's an education. The best sex tip I ever picked up from reading erotica was in a 'True Confessions' type of column in a magazine. The writer said she'd recently discovered the 'Bowling Ball Grip', which involved her being on all fours, while her man placed his thumb in her butt and his two middle fingers in her vagina; he then rubbed the fingers and thumb together to massage the connecting wall. I've tried it a few times since and it's been rather successful.

Tim, 39

I intended to return the favour and wasn't taking no for an answer. I tore at David's combats, freeing his delicious dick. I really do love that scent, that taste – each man with his own unique, musky blend. David had shaved his balls and I lapped all around them like a hungry cat at a bowl of milk, then I took each one in my mouth, rolling my tongue around them. My fist, slick with my saliva, pumped the head of his dick, then my mouth followed suit, furiously bobbing up and down as David's moans caused the dampness in my knickers to spread.

'I'm gonna come,' he warned, and I took his cock out of my mouth and directed his spray over my open lips, licking in his juices while he watched.

Later, as the plane landed, Neil woke up. I wondered if he'd ever believe David, as I felt sure David would tell him, but my curiosity was only passing. As the plane doors opened, I said it was nice to meet them, but I had to dash. Another lie. I just didn't want to sully a hot memory with small talk.

'Thanks for travelling with us,' said the smiling air steward as I skipped off the plane.

'The pleasure was all mine.'

Real Sex
Equality Erotica

The Sexual Life of Catherine M. by Catherine Millet has gone down in history as the most explicit book about sex ever written by a woman; a forerunner to the many sexual memoirs we see from women writers today, this is the original groundbreaker. What I love is the fact that Catherine looks at sex the same way a man does, enjoying sexual encounters (the wilder the better) with as many people as possible, never experiencing any guilt. The text is full of tips, and reading this at bedtime is foreplay in itself.

Joanna, 35

The Power of Three

I stood up and pulled off my top, slipped my skirt over my high-heeled shoes and unclasped my bra, letting my breasts fall. Then I sat down, parting my thighs ever so slightly, and watched as their eyes shifted to gaze at my black lace knickers.

'Take off your clothes,' I said, trying to sound braver than I felt. And as easy as that, I had two naked men in my room. Looking at their different forms, I began to wonder how the men would feel inside me, how they would differ, and my anxiety was quickly replaced with sexual tension.

I stood up and turned to kiss Lewis, enjoying his skilful lips and tongue on mine as Danny pressed his body to my back, his erection against my buttocks and his fingers twisting my nipples. My lovers then carefully laid me down on the double bed, Lewis's hand slipping under my lacy underwear and parting my pink wet lips as I arched my back with pleasure. But it was Danny who pulled off my knickers, licking my clit as he did so. Lewis – it must have been Lewis – then stroked my aching passage, twirling his fingers inside me, making me cry out as sex pulsed through my veins. Already I was coming, bucking my hips as waves of release flowed over me, but the night was still young.

'How very rude of me,' I murmured, smiling as I repositioned myself, kneeling on the floor, two beautiful cocks now in my eye-line. I wondered how to please both.

Taking a deep breath, I began to run my tongue over and around the head of one, while rhythmically sliding my hand up and down the other, amazed by the delicacy of the skins overlaying their hard shafts.

I began to work in earnest, taking the head of Lewis's cock in my mouth, and then Danny's, gradually taking them deeper. I raised my body up, then rubbed the shiny, swollen heads over my breasts, my nipples hardening to announce my arousal. Then I took each man in turn into my throat until I could feel the familiar swell, the rush to climax.

'Not just yet, boys,' I said, and laid Danny down on the bed, kissing my way up his body as I straddled him, presenting my enticing derrière to Lewis. I felt Lewis's hands firmly grip my hips and a cold trickle of lube spread over me, then he gently nudged his way inside.

I pushed back on to Lewis as he filled me up, then let out a moan of ecstasy as Danny pushed up between my wet lips and began to fuck me.

They took me in earnest, driving sweet pleasure deep into me. I rose and fell softly at first, then faster as I enjoyed how tightly I held each of them inside me. Lewis's warm chest pressed against my back; Danny's hands squeezed my heavy breasts, and my convulsing orgasm triggered theirs.

Stretched out in the afterglow, Danny nuzzling my chest, Lewis resting his head on my shoulder, I began to laugh. And then we were all laughing, feeling like we must surely have just discovered the true joy of sex.

The Night Nina and Olivia Met

Back in Nina's bedroom, their two pussies slide together, a perfect match of fragrance – musk and sweetness. Olivia crushes Nina's generous tits together, so she can reach both nipples with one long lick. She's never tasted any pussy but her own, but she's sure Nina's will be melt-in-the-mouth tasty. She can tell from Nina's scent – it's making her hungry.

They feel like two teenagers doing it for the first time; they wriggle and slide on top, underneath, on top again. Sometimes Olivia feels more like the boy as she pins Nina's hands above her head, straddling her on the bed and rubbing against her; other times Nina takes control, wrestles herself up, throws Olivia on her back and yanks her legs wide apart, so she can push her face there. This isn't Nina's first time, and she knows exactly what she wants.

Both slick with sweat, their bodies twist around until their mouths are open wide at each other's shining pink slits, sucking and prodding and demanding more. Their only noises are high giggles and deep grunts and the 'smack, smack' sound of wet flesh on wet flesh.

Olivia passes Nina a black strap-on – a huge one. It fits round Nina's waist like it's tailor-made, the weight pressing on to her pubic bone. She stands with her legs wide apart, one hand resting on that cock – her cock! – the other between Olivia's legs as she lies there now, spread-eagled and passive.

Nina stands over her momentarily submissive partner and rams her hard cock into her and it's a whole new world. Olivia thrusts back and moans, and Nina bucks and bucks, up on her knees with Olivia's legs wrapped around her. Nina feels the base of the hard rubber rock press back against her clit and watches Olivia's hips piston back and forth in rhythm, her head thrown back and mouth gaping, eyes unfocused. She understands why male porn stars always look so smug.

Moaning loudly now, Olivia is spiralling towards orgasm, going somewhere the big fake cock, lovely though it is, can't take Nina, so Nina has to take her hand off Olivia's smooth belly and slide it beneath the strap-on to reach her own swollen clit. She rubs and rocks herself to the same place, playing catch-up with the X-rated figure on the duvet in front of her, who seems to be impaled on the black stick like a human sex lollipop.

As Nina comes, she yanks her fake cock out, bends forwards and, through her own moans, puts her still-hungry mouth over Olivia's slick pussy and sucks and sucks and sucks the hot juice out of her.

Later, when Nina walks home, her pussy is bruising and aching from the great big fake cock; her knees are scraped and the muscles in her shoulders feel torn from holding herself up over the delicious Olivia, but despite all these things – and because of them – she has never felt better.

Real Sex
Girls Who Like Girls' Books

I'm married and have never been with a woman in my life, but my best friend is a lesbian and she lent me some books. I used to be a strictly *Black Lace* sort of girl, but lesbian erotica is hot! I'd always wondered how, exactly, women have sex with each other and now I know. Sometimes, when my hubby's going down on me I imagine his tongue is one of the character's tongues I've just read about. He's fine with it – I've told him and he says it turns him on, so everyone's a winner in my (erotic lesbian) book! My current favourite is *Best Lesbian Erotica 2008* edited by Tristan Taormino – thank you, Tristan!

Jodie, 27

Two Men and a Tub

Young men bathing outside was not considered unusual. Few people could afford indoor baths and the climate was so amenable that it was no hardship to sluice down in the yard with a few buckets of cold water and a bar of cracked soap. What was unusual was that this particular young man was watched, almost inadvertently, by another.

Paolo wasn't just some dirty old man. He wasn't even old – he was young, healthy and happily married to a pretty young woman called Elena. He wasn't sexually starved either – Elena had a hearty appetite for his dark thighs against her own burnt-sugar ones. Which was why he was so shocked by the way his body responded to the sight of his new neighbour washing in the yard.

He was sitting on the windowsill, sneakily reading one of Elena's lurid melodramas – the kind that he was so disapproving of in her presence. The rebels had just made off with the gypsy king's daughter, slung over the pommel of the rebel leader's saddle, and Paolo looked up from the purloined book, gazing out of the window as he wondered how Elena would look hanging sideways off a horse. It was then that he caught sight of the naked man in the yard next door.

He couldn't have been much older than twenty; tanned, Hispanic and muscled like a manual labourer. He poured the bucket of water over his head and shook like a dog, droplets of water catching the sun as they fanned outwards from his body. The glitter of the South American rays on the flying water caught Paolo's attention. He noted the uninhibited, animal quality to the man's movements as he began to lather up the soap and rub it over his body. His skin was the same brown sugar colour as Elena's, with the same burnished glow, and Paolo remembered how Elena's body looked covered with beads of water when she bathed in her beloved tin bath. He felt a stiffening and a heat in his trousers, and blushed at how this man had made it come about. He shot a look of hatred and embarrassment at the oblivious bather.

The young man was covered in creamy suds, rubbing his hands vigorously over his arms and legs. As Paolo watched the man's tightly knotted muscles and sinews flex as he bent and twisted, he felt his hardness increase and, momentarily, wondered how it would feel to touch those contoured, wet thighs. He just as quickly tried to banish the thought from his mind, but it would not go. A tiny part of Paolo wanted those thoughts, enjoyed thinking about how those powerful bronze hands would feel on his own chocolate body. How those hands would treat his now-prominent erection. Would they be harder, firmer than Elena's? Surely they would. Would it feel good?

Paolo struggled with himself again. This was wrong. He'd never had feelings for other men. He'd bathed naked with men before, swimming in the river or standing under open showers after football games. He'd never felt even a flicker of curiosity. And yet here he was, rock hard, sweating under his cotton shirt at the sight of this young man.

The man began to carefully wash his penis, treating it as gently as if it were a fragile bird that might expire. Paolo gave in and pulled his trousers and pants down round his ankles. Wetting his hand, he slid it up and down his blue-black shaft, groaning softly at the intensity of the feeling. The man in the courtyard stood up, displaying his strong, broad back, golden and smooth, streaked with white lather.

Paolo – almost beyond guilt now – imagined adding his own pearly come to the man's torso. He wanted the man to take his – Paolo's – throbbing and burning cock, place it between those full, almost feminine, lips and feel the softness of his wet, silky, soothing tongue. Would he be able to take more than Elena? Let Paolo insert his entire length in his mouth? Paolo felt a warmth like molten copper spread through his veins – delicious, irresistible, yet too strong to bear with comfort. He cried out softly, his cock desperate for release as he pumped with his tightening hand, arching his back against the wall as he strove towards orgasm.

As the young Hispanic man rubbed his body dry with a worn blue towel, Paolo imagined sinking between those high buttocks and, at the thought of the two powerful male bodies embracing, two pairs of strong hands stroking and grabbing at each other, two pairs of pert, boyish bums and two hard and eager cocks, he came, electricity singing in his nerves, his mouth dry from his silent cries.

Later that night Paolo made love to Elena like it was their very first time.

Real Sex
Sharing Shorts

You can tell a lot about a lover's fantasies from the sort of erotica they respond to. I like to read Anaïs Nin. *Delta of Venus* is her best collection of erotic stories – the little slices of sexual life cover all kinds of uncommon scenarios from flashing on public transport in 'Manuel' to kinky games of voyeurism in 'The Veiled Woman' (my favourite – and a story I'd actually like to act out one day). Sharing short stories is also a sexy way to spend time on the phone with a long-distance lover, to keep your fires burning.

Lucia, 31

Mixing Business and Pleasure

Angela works on the floor above me. Marketing; not my department. But I always hear about her. Everyone talks about Angela. Terrible Angela. What has she done this time? Today she got so angry, she shouted at a client on the phone and lost the account.

I think about how much trouble she ought to be in for that. I play squash with her line manager sometimes. We always talk about Angela. She has ways. Charm. She called up that client. Made it good. Had his favourite chocolate truffles sent over. By the time Richard called her into his office for a talking to, it was all sorted, she said. But she offered to suck Richard off for good measure, he adds, making me miss my shot as my dick swells in my pants. She did it too, licking him slowly at first, then faster and faster. She swallowed his juices as though they were ambrosia.

After hearing about that from Richard, hiding my arousal with breathlessness, I fist my cock in the shower and think about what a dirty minx she is. The next morning, in the toilets at work, I have my hand on my cock again. We have unisex toilets – an idea some bright spark thought was cool a few years ago – which means I overhear all kinds of salacious talk while I'm locked in the far cubicle. I think the two women I'm listening to are called Trudy and Tricia. The first one, the one with the flattest estuary vowels, says, 'That's not the half of it. Yeah, she sucked him off in his office, but then they went home together.'

'They fucked?' I hear the second voice whisper.

'Yup. Richard told Eric in Marketing. But that's not all . . . '

'Oh God,' says the second voice, and I echo the sentiment. Bad, bad Angela. My cock is harder now, jutting out of my flies. I coil my fingers around it and all I can think of is Angela getting what she deserves. I know what bad girls get. I'm lost in a fantasy about Angela bent over my lap. Her hands are tied behind her back and she's rubbing herself on my erection. I spank her. Harder and harder. I push her off my lap and make her suck my hard cock. Then I push her off and shove her down on the floor. I hold her by her bound wrists and ram myself into her from behind. She's soaking wet and her well-spanked arse is burning hot against my flesh.

Panting, I suddenly let go of my cock. I don't want to come too soon.

Outside, estuary vowels says, 'And you know what?' Her voice is more unctuous than ever. 'She was crap. Apparently Angela was crap in bed. Lazy, Richard told Eric. Just lay there and let him do all the work.'

My dick is still in my hand. But it's suddenly going soft. What? I just don't believe it. She'd never . . . Angela would never be . . .

Later that morning, I find some flimsy excuse to have Angela come to my office. When I call her in, she looks flustered. I'm hard under my desk. Angela's curly blonde hair is askew. She's such a floozy. Her cock-sucking mouth is too pink and so obvious. I swallow. And then she smirks at me. 'What do you want?' she says.

'You fucked Richard,' I say, sternly.

'So?' She's doing a good job of faking nonchalance, but I can see right through her. Her cheeks tinge pink. Caught out.

'I heard you were selfish in bed.'

Now she's genuinely flustered. 'What? No way. I did everything he asked. Just like you told me. I obeyed him as if he were you.' I frown at her and she looks worried. 'I swear. I did just what you wanted. What you liked. I can't believe he said that.' The pink in her cheeks is rising, and I know now it's only partly embarrassment, part arousal. She loves this whole sordid game.

'He didn't. But I overheard some rather interesting gossip.' I hold up a hand and pat the desk in front of me.

'What? Here in your office?' But she's already moving into position. 'I knew it,' she says, bending over the desk and gripping the far edge as I pick up a ruler. 'You're jealous.'

'Maybe I am.' I push up her skirt. She doesn't wear knickers. That's one of my rules. I shove two fingers right into her. She's so wet. I pull out again and she moans. I take a step back, raising the ruler in the air.

She laughs. 'I said you would be . . . ' She cuts off abruptly as I bring the ruler down across her bottom. 'People might hear,' she whispers. She has a point. I reach around and place a wad of Post-Its between her smooth, pearly teeth, then proceed to create a series of corset-like lines across the ample cleavage of her arse with my ruler. As I watch the red welts rise, I roughly penetrate my masterpiece, savagely thrusting until I can feel the ripples of her orgasm grip me. Bad, bad Angela. She just can't get enough.

Real Sex
BDSM Bible

Any man or woman whose fantasises include elements of sado-masochism should read *Story of O* by the French woman who wrote under the name Pauline Réague. The central character, O, is a willing sex slave who gives her permission to be trained to service several men in a variety of twisted ways. The famous author Graham Greene said it was a rare thing: a porno book that was well written without a trace of obscenity. I don't practise the lifestyle, but I read a lot of BDSM books for sexual escapism, and I still haven't come across one that's better than this.

Mark, 42

Exercise B

Role-play Rehearsal – Personalised Erotica, Starring You!

Now you've tried reading other people's stories, I'd like to draw you into a story of your own. Putting yourself in the roles of the lead characters lets you dip a toe in the waters of different fantasy scenarios. If you like what you feel, you can create a story together as a rehearsal for real role play.

To demonstrate this, I've selected a piece of erotica about a lap dancer and a customer that you can also act out at home, using your lounge as the club and your bedroom as the elusive 'VIPs Only' room. You'll also need to dress for the part, pick a suitable soundtrack and invest in a bottle of flavoured lube.

First, in the spaces provided, fill in your own names; men, your name goes on the solid lines that look like this: _____; ladies, your name goes on the broken lines that look like this: ....

Once all the spaces are filled, nominate a narrator to read the story out loud, then focus on actually being the characters in your mind. At the end of today's lesson, feel free to enact your very own dramatisation.

Your Story: The Lap of Luxury

_____ watched .... from across the room. As he took in the small waist, tight round buttocks and perfect legs, he felt his cock give an involuntary spasm and harden.

A sheer, delicate dress clung to .... 's body, the neckline cut low to reveal her welcoming cleavage. Sitting in the shadows, _____ watched as .... gyrated around the stage, ignoring the crowd, listening instead to the music, stroking her breasts and flicking her luscious hair wildly. _____ wished she would gyrate on his cock in the same fashion, but he was painfully aware of the fact that she ignored him every time he came here.

As the song ended, instead of exiting stage left as she usually did, ... strutted down the steps and into the crowd, heading,

_____ thought, in his direction. Surely he must be mistaken, but heat prickled the back of his neck anyway, and his dick grew harder.

'Would you like to dance?' .... purred. _____ looked around to make sure she really was speaking to him. 'I've seen you watching me, and I don't just mean today,' she continued, 'but the thing is I've been watching you too.'

Taking _____ by the hand, ... drew him towards a door marked 'VIPS ONLY' and keyed in an entry code. The door opened and inside the candlelit room _____ could see a double bed and a dressing table scattered with lubricants and sex toys. .... turned to look at him as she slipped her dress over her shoulders, letting it fall to the floor to reveal her unashamed nakedness.

'How much?' he croaked, throat dry with excitement, quite sure he couldn't afford what he could see before him.

.... shook her head. 'This one's on me,' she said, smiling as she uncapped an ornate bottle of lube and slowly trickled the glistening fluid over her hard, pert nipples. 'Cherry flavour,' she said. 'You like cherries?'

.... gently pushed _____ on to the bed, so he was sitting in front of her, then fed her nipples into his already open mouth, one at a time, after tracing the tip of each around his lips. He could taste the cherry ... cherry-flavoured lap dancer.

'I want your cock,' whispered .... Reaching down she found the solid mass of his erection, then quickly unbuttoned his trousers and pushed him back further so she could free his manhood from the constraints of his boxer shorts. His swollen dick sprang from beneath the fabric, begging to be touched, engulfed, fucked. First, a cold trail of lube was delicately coiled around the head – every second a sweet torment. Then .... 's tongue; hot, twirling, fluttering, divine.

Sliding up his sweat- and lube-drenched body, ... 's breasts reached _____'s cock, and sandwiched tightly between them he bucked up as she lapped at the protruding head.

Sensing he was nearing the edge of orgasm, ... slowed the pace with one long, hard suck of his dick, as she plunged her finger inside the warm well of her pussy. 'See how wet I am?' she asked, almost innocently, as she brought her finger to his mouth for tasting. Then she straddled him, and at last he felt the velvet of her folds above his face. Sucking, licking and flicking, he focused his tongue on the sweet, juicy bud of her clit, hooking three strong fingers inside her, pulling her sex down to him. Now it was .... who found herself close to climax.

She pulled away and moved down his torso, pausing to hover above the erection he held upright for her, her dripping opening just touching the tip of his cock. Their eyes locked. Their breaths were held. Intense, unadulterated anticipation. Then whoosh! Juices splashed, breasts bounced, heartbeats quickened, blood surged through their veins, and then come, so much come, his, hers, hot and sticky, the scent filling the air.

'Everything OK in there?' a bouncer called through the door.

'Er . . . yeah, thanks . . . everything's great. Be out in a minute.' _____ composed herself. Within seconds she'd slipped her dress back on and pulled up and refastened _____'s trousers. Before turning to leave, she knelt over him and planted a kiss on his mouth, briefly tasting herself there.

'Take a few minutes if you need to,' she smiled. 'Oh, and I shouldn't have to tell you this, but what we just did – it never happened.'

Exercise C
Sexual Ad Lib and Improvisation – Greater Fluency in the Language of Lust

Now you've tasted the language of sex, it's time to get fluent. This means drawing on your own imagination to talk dirty, so you can 'wax physical' any time you like without needing to follow a script. But first, I need you to discuss your own personal preferences when it comes to sex vocab. It's crucial that you both know which words are likely to turn each other on or off.

Personally, I don't get turned on by the term 'pussy'. It reminds me of family pets. I prefer – and please look away, if you're easily offended – 'cunt'. This controversial term is not to everyone's taste; I rarely use it in print, and this is the only time you'll see it in this book, but, to me, it's sexy, loaded with power and strength.

Now tell each other which words work for you and which don't. Write them down for memory's sake in the grid provided. Then you'll be ready to move on to the next part of this exercise.

Your Sex Vocab

His turn-on words

_____

_____

_____

_____

_____

Her turn-on words

_____

_____

_____

_____

_____

His turn-off words

_____

_____

_____

_____

_____

Her turn-off words

_____

_____

_____

_____

_____

Real Sex
What a Boon!

I recently read *The Director's Wife* by Lindsay Armstrong. It's a Mills & Boon book, so the focus wasn't all on the sex, but there was a scene in which the director of the title and his wife got steamy on his yacht. In the dark of night, they're sharing a hot shower on deck and get caught in the headlights of another boat. This scene really got me going because of the unusual alfresco setting and the element of being caught. Hot follow-up fantasies ahoy!

Emilie, 25

In the grid below, you'll see a selection of characters, venues and props. Together, pick one from column one, two from column two and three from column three. These characters, locations and aids will form the basis of your ad-libbed sexual scenario. Lie back, relax and take turns to tell mini chapters of your story based on the elements you've selected – the aim is to make the story so sexy that you can't keep your hands off each other.

For example, you could pick: police officer and criminal, a forest and a cell, and a camera, handcuffs and dildo (think truncheon). With the guy in the police officer role, he could catch the female criminal. Her crime? Masturbating in a public place, the forest. The police officer could then take photos with his camera for evidence, then escort the handcuffed prisoner to the cell and punish her with his 'truncheon' when no one's looking.

Characters (select one)	Locations (select two)	Props (select three)
○ Yourselves	○ An office	○ Dildo
○ Teacher and pupil	○ A cell or dungeon	○ Telephone
○ Photographer and nude model	○ Your bedroom	○ Whip / spanking paddle
○ Doctor and patient	○ A hotel	○ Handcuffs/wrist binds
○ High-class escort and client	○ A beach	○ Lubricant
○ Burglar/kidnapper and victim	○ Public transport	○ Vibrator
○ Phone-sex operator and caller	○ A car	○ Camera
○ Police officer and criminal	○ A toilet	○ Butt plug
○ Dominatrix and sex slave	○ A forest	○ Penis ring
○ Boss and personal assistant	○ A swingers' club	○ Chocolate body paint

By the time you've completed this exercise you should feel more comfortable talking before and during sex. It will take the investment of time and practice to be able to spin red-hot, erotic scenarios off the top of your head, and it's worth doing, but most people don't need to hear a monologue. If you can say, 'Yes, that feels so hot' and 'Oh yeah, harder/ faster' without dying of embarrassment, you're on the right track.

Later today, you'll also learn how to talk about sex after the fact – those awkward conversations that no one really wants to have about sexual issues, but which crop up in every relationship. Before that though, let's take a look at porn.

Extra-curricular Activity
Verbal foreplay

Today, you've worked out how to harness the power of words as a sexual stimulant to be used as foreplay or an orgasm trigger. Words are like a vibrator for the brain, and, better still, they can be used just about anywhere. Try texting or emailing sexplicit messages to your lover – sent in sequence over the course of a day, this will guarantee that they come home to you in the mood for lust. Or try whispering something naughty in a lover's ear at an inappropriate time and place (I'm thinking a restaurant when you're having dinner, rather than a funeral or when you're at a wake).

Exercise D

The Truth About Porn Films – What X-rated Movies Can Do For You

First of all, let's bust some myths about porn films. In a study where participants' heart rates were monitored for levels of arousal, both men and women were made to watch various scenes from porn films. The results showed that the physical responses were no different in men than they were in women, even for those women who said they didn't get off on porn. It was concluded that while some viewers may feel uncomfortable about certain aspects of pornography, and that this may overshadow the benefits of being aroused by it, seeing sexual images pumps blood to our genitals. In other words, whether we like it or not, it turns us on.

Also, for the record, I've never – repeat never – known a woman recommend a porn film to me because it had a great storyline. Jerry Barnett, a friend of mine who runs StrictlyBroadband.com, the UK's leading adult film site, can, at any given time, list the most popular films currently being viewed by men and women on his site. At the time of going to press, *Bisexual Encounters of the Exxxtreme Kind* and *The World's Biggest Gangbang* were in the ladies' top ten – and, let me tell you, storylines don't feature in either.

Now we've got that cleared up, it's time for you to talk about how you both *really* feel about porn. To break the ice, tick the box next to each of the following statements that applies to you, then read on for my responses, as you discuss these issues openly and without recrimination.

Him	Her	
☐	☐	I'm worried my partner finds the actors more attractive than me.
☐	☐	I think the orgasms look fake and the sex techniques are poor.
☐	☐	I feel the actors are being exploited.
☐	☐	I don't find the actors attractive enough to get turned on.
☐	☐	I don't want to watch porn with my partner; I prefer to watch alone.
☐	☐	I don't want my partner to watch porn without me.
☐	☐	I don't like that my partner is secretive about watching porn.
☐	☐	Watching porn makes me feel embarrassed and self-conscious.

Your Issues Addressed

I'm worried my partner finds the actors more attractive than me

I know I'm not the first woman and I won't be the last to feel intimidated by porn stars – and I'm 100 per cent sure it's no different for men when a strapping Adonis with 10 inches swinging between his legs enters a scene. The most prolific porn stars, the ones we see most often, got to where they are today because their sex organs look good on camera: the men have insanely large members that never seem to go soft and the women have perfectly symmetrical, neat and tidy labia, palatable pink anal cavities and, unlike the rest of the female population, they don't seem to suffer from shaving rashes and ingrown hairs.

This unattainable perfection is what turns some men and women on, and if you're both secure in your own skin and comfortable seeing physical perfection paraded in front of you, go ahead and soak it up. That's what it's there for: your sexual gratification. Think of the actors as servants for your desires or pretty sexual accessories, like designer sex toys.

However, when one of you doesn't feel comfortable, it's time to look at making some compromises: you can either agree to watch porn separately or you can change the sort of porn you watch. Professional films advertising 'natural' actors feature more regular-looking stars with stretch marks, cellulite, smaller penises and fewer implants. Amateur porn films *are* made by regular **people** and you'll see everything from spotty bottoms to family photos **on shelves**. Too far? Watch a selection and find out where your preference **lies**.

I think the orgasms look fake and the sex techniques are poor

They often are. When making porn films, most directors have a male market in mind. As a result, you're likely to see a lot of what I call 'porn cunnilingus', or – change a couple of letters to get the more accurate description – poor cunnilingus. The male actor will hold his face as far away from his co-star's genitals as possible, then poke out his tongue and flick it. This allows the camera to get up close to the action, but every woman knows that what the co-star really wants is for him to bury his face between her legs like he's ducking for apples. Likewise, during penetrative sex, thrusts are long and drawn out and clitoral contact is minimal. Again, this allows for better camera angles, but it's hard to be convinced (as a woman, at least) when said co-star suddenly starts convulsing in orgasm after three of these long strokes.

The key to enjoying this sort of porn is not to critique it, but to take a leap of faith and let your own private fantasies entwine with the show. If you can't do this, change your porn. Look for films by female porn directors such as Anna Span, where more attention is given to technique; watch amateur porn, where the sex is real and so the techniques work (at least for the couple on the screen); or get yourself a camcorder and make your own porn.

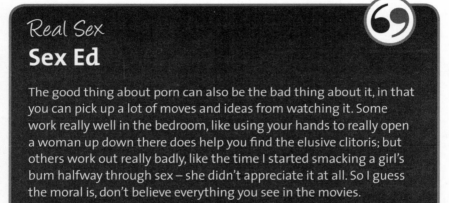

Real Sex
Sex Ed

The good thing about porn can also be the bad thing about it, in that you can pick up a lot of moves and ideas from watching it. Some work really well in the bedroom, like using your hands to really open a woman up down there does help you find the elusive clitoris; but others work out really badly, like the time I started smacking a girl's bum halfway through sex – she didn't appreciate it at all. So I guess the moral is, don't believe everything you see in the movies.

Ben, 25

I feel the actors are being exploited

As porn has become more mainstream, a lot of progress has been made in preventing the mistreatment of actors. However, it would be foolish to think exploitation has been wiped out completely. Again, watching amateur porn can help here. When there's no money changing hands, there's less chance of behind-the-scenes exploitation. On free websites like YouPorn.com the public upload their own private films – not for profit, but because they enjoy being watched. Sure, some of the regulars are wannabe porn stars, putting together a portfolio, but a lot of people just get off on you getting off on them. What a great free exchange!

If you're into glossier porn, select films featuring the most powerful women in porn – actresses like Tera Patrick, who also runs her own agency that stipulates and ensures actors are treated with respect, and Jenna Jameson, worth an estimated 30 million dollars, who runs her own production company, stars in her own films and is way beyond ever being exploited.

I don't find the actors attractive enough to get turned on

Guys, can you look away now, please . . . Ladies, I think there's a bit of a conspiracy going on in a lot of porn films, in that the women are almost always a lot better looking than the men (which is why I'm addressing this issue with you, rather than your partners). It seems that while male porn directors purposely pick out large and resilient penises, they also deliberately opt for less than attractive faces. The fact is, they don't want the guy's face to attract anything. All attention is directed to the women in each scene, and, that way, the male viewer doesn't feel in competition with the actor. Great for male viewers; not so great for females.

To get a fair crack at the eye candy, pick porn made by female directors, and for solo sex sessions, check out gay porn: the men are far more beautiful because they're cast for their face as well as their foot-long schlongs, the sex is raw and intriguing and it's an amazing insight into male sexuality. I'm guessing most bristling heterosexual men wouldn't want to share the experience with you – but then maybe you don't want to watch the likes of the stunning Ms Tera Patrick with him?

I don't want to watch porn with my partner; I prefer to watch alone

If your partner has issues with you watching porn alone, ask them why and share your reasons for wanting to watch porn alone. Perhaps you just want to have some sex time that's purely about you; perhaps you'd feel jealous about your partner getting turned on by something that isn't you; or maybe you feel your partner wouldn't enjoy the show and that would detract from your enjoyment. Whatever your reasons, be honest with yourself, as well as your partner, and, wherever possible, offer reassurance en route to finding a resolution. Maybe you could share some screenings and not others?

I don't want my partner to watch porn without me

Our masturbation habits shouldn't be policed by our partners. Whether we use toys, sexual fantasises (which are just an internal, self-directed sort of porn, anyway) or real porn, we should be able to do so without feeling guilty.

Extra-curricular Activity

Bonkbusters

Having trouble finding any porn film to suit your taste? Maybe a mainstream film with extra-hot sex scenes would be better for you. Here are five that became famous for their explicit content:

- *The Postman Always Rings Twice* (1981) Jack Nicholson and Jessica Lange show us how it's really done on the kitchen table with oral sex and hand-jobs for her and a straddling finale!

- *Bound* (1996) Intensely erotic girl-on-girl action with Jennifer Tilly and Gina Gershon.

- *Secretary* (2002) James Spader and Maggie Gyllenhaal demonstrate sexual power play between boss and secretary.

- *Last Tango In Paris* (1972) Marlon Brando famously uses butter as his choice of lubricant in a brutal anal-sex scene with co-star Maria Schneider.

- *Blue Velvet* (1986) Voyeur Kyle MacLachlan watches from another room, while Isabella Rossellini takes part in extreme sex acts with Dennis Hopper.

First, examine your reasons for feeling this way and discuss them with your partner. Often people can feel jealous of a lover's porn habit, and that jealousy often springs from low self-esteem and feelings of insecurity. In short, when you love yourself you're less likely to think, He's/she's watching those actors because I'm too short/fat/ugly to look at.

Don't pretend to like porn just because a partner does, either. Porn is not for everyone, and it's easy to spot a faker. If you really want to watch adult films together, first invest time into finding some that *you* like and only then share them with your lover. If you get off on them, you partner will get off on seeing you aroused. But don't be offended if your lover still likes to watch films alone. It only becomes a problem if their arousal depends on it and their view of sex becomes so distorted that they're disappointed when real lovemaking doesn't live up to the screen version.

I don't like that my partner is secretive about watching porn

I know a lot of men who (and a few women) who hide their porn stash. This is part habit (after growing up having to hide porn from our parents) and part negative conditioning. If your partner has been scolded by previous lovers for keeping porn, they're more likely to hide it in the future.

The key to bringing a lover's porn out into the open is to demonstrate an open mind. When you happen upon a partner's stash, don't get angry because they've been keeping something from you; instead say, 'Hey, I stumbled across your *Shaving Ryan's Privates* – it looks like a fun DVD. Can I borrow it?' You might not enjoy it, but at least the issue is no longer taboo, and this could lead to seeing more films together that you do enjoy.

Real Sex
When Porn Hurts

I found my boyfriend's porn magazine down behind the back of our wardrobe. It actually made me feel physically sick – not because of the content, it was actually pretty tame compared to the sort of weird things that get emailed around the Internet – but because I'd had no idea that he owned one. I felt like he'd lied. In fact, I felt like he'd been unfaithful. I looked at the women in the mag and compared myself to them and felt so ugly. I accept that everyone fantasises about other people, but it's harder when you get to see a picture of the other person's face. I guess if Justin Timberlake did nude shoots, I'd be hiding them down the back of the wardrobe too, and I just have to remember that – and, of course, the fact that's there's actually no emotional connection between me and Justin – whenever I feel jealousy over what my boyfriend fantasises about. It's a tough lesson to learn though.

Lisa, 26

Watching porn makes me feel embarrassed and self-conscious

Until you're actually aroused, all porn looks pretty ridiculous. Allow yourself time to catch up with the seemingly ever-ready actors you're watching and expect to laugh at first. A few giggles makes great foreplay!

Once you're feeling a little hot under the collar, initiate a little session of your own, while the porn is playing in the background. You could go down on your partner, or ask them to go down on you, while you continue to watch the film; or you could get into a position where you can both watch, such as doggy-style, her sitting on his lap or reverse cowgirl (the standard woman-on-top position, but where she faces away from him).

Extra-curricular Activity
Porn games

To make watching porn more interesting, agree to re-enact each of your favourite scenes from a film when you're done watching it. If the scene has more than two characters in it, improvise third parties using dildos and masturbation sleeves.

If a film has excessive cheesy dialogue, turn it to your advantage by picking out the most clichéd word or phrase – 'big' and 'hard' are usually safe bets – and then each strip off another item of clothing whenever an actor says that word. You'll soon both be naked and too busy soaking up each other to care about how bad the film is.

Exercise E
The Sex Confessional – Transferring Your Talking Skills to Sexual Issues

Now, all that remains today is for me to guide you through the sort of sex conversations that most people dread: the ones where you need to raise any problems you feel you're having. It's essential that you learn to do this, as all couples, at some point in their relationships, will experience issues that need ironing out, and the only way to do this is through candid and well-considered discussion.

Remember, having occasional problems in the bedroom does not indicate a doomed relationship – but not being able to talk about them does. Once you've completed this exercise, you'll be able to face your fear of awkward sex talks and feel confident talking openly about any issues you have.

Right now, having completed Days One to Six of my plan, chances are you're feeling better about your sex life than you have done in ages. And if there's absolutely nothing niggling either of you, move on – but remember, this exercise is always here for you at any time you may need it in the future.

If there is ever something you need to get off your chest, here are the five golden rules to having that all-important chat:

1. Think about the reasons behind the issue. Our sex likes and dislikes are unique to us and evolve for a number of reasons – not all of them involving the partner we're with. Our bodies – and our erogenous zones – change over time, so what turns us on one month, may lose its appeal the next, simply because of physical changes. Psychologically, our religion, previous sexual history and upbringing can also affect how we view sex.

Take whatever issue you have and analyse it. For example, perhaps you want sex more often. If so, ask yourself why: as a couple do you rarely have sex? Or is it because you have a higher-than-average libido? Or is it because getting more sex makes you feel more loved? If it's the latter, are there other ways your partner can show you love, and are there ways you can learn to feel more secure in yourself without using sex as an emotional prop? If you have a higher libido than your partner's, could more frequent masturbation sessions for you balance out your sex drives? If you have sex very rarely, what are the reasons?

Think long and hard about these reasons because knowing the root cause of an issue will help you reach the right solution. In severe cases, tailored counselling sessions with a sex therapist may be called for, but in most instances, open, candid communication with your lover will be enough to resolve problems, so long as you adhere to these five golden rules.

2. Choose the right moment to broach an issue. Never bring up sex issues in the heat of an argument. This may seem like an obvious statement, but so many people – especially those who have been harbouring resentment over something they've been unable to talk about – do just that. Which leads me to my next point: never harbour issues. As soon as you feel uncomfortable about something, pledge to raise the issue at the first suitable moment, because the longer it festers, the bigger it will seem and the more hurt your partner will be that you withheld the information. But what is a suitable moment? That varies from couple to couple. Some people prefer to talk about sex in the bedroom, immediately after sex when still wrapped in each other's arms, flooded with relaxing post-sex hormones. This can work well in certain instances. For example, if you feel you aren't having sex as often as you'd like, you could say, 'Wow, I really enjoyed that; I'd like to make more time to do it more often – would you?' Other couples prefer to keep sex problems out of the bedroom, and, in reality, you can talk just about anywhere you feel comfortable and have privacy with no distractions (sharing a bath together, over a nice meal at home or a picnic in a park, perhaps, or cuddled up on the sofa, TV switched off). Whichever environment you opt for, avoid drinking to help you relax (one glass is OK, but after that it's just as likely to make you less focused or even argumentative) and try to maintain some physical contact – either holding hands, cuddling or stroking each other – so your body language remains positive.

3. Never begin with 'You . . . ' This sets up an accusatory tone, so think carefully before you speak. Instead of saying, 'You never pay me any compliments', say, 'Sometimes I feel a little insecure and I'd love to hear what you find sexy about me'.

4. Try to include a compliment with your request. Flattery may not get you everywhere, but it will get you a damn sight further than a complaint. For example, instead of saying, 'You never go down on me', say, 'You're so good with your tongue – I'd love more oral sex'.

5. Try to suggest a solution to your issue. Bringing up problems can seem negative or nagging if there's no solution available, so before bringing up an issue, also think about how you'd like to try to solve it. Rather than saying, 'You never initiate sex', you could say, 'I feel like I'm a little too controlling in the bedroom, and I'd like to try being tied up to see how it feels'.

With these rules in mind, take turns to reveal something that's been playing on your mind. It could be that a particular move your partner is so proud of doesn't really work for you; or perhaps you'd like to try sex in a new location; or maybe you want a little more romance with your sex. Whatever your issue, if you follow the five rules above, you should be able to express yourself without causing offence.

At the same time, appreciate that your partner may have needs that aren't being met or issues they want to discuss. That isn't necessarily a reflection on you, but it *is* something that you need to know about. Allow them to feel safe and comfortable sharing their thoughts, listen to what they have to say and remember: addressing their issues isn't just about improving *their* sex life, it's about improving *yours* too. You're in this together, after all.

By following today's lessons you've learnt how to get your tongue around sex! You've read erotica out loud, personalised a story you can act out as role play, shared fresh fantasies of your own and ascertained exactly where you both stand on porn – that's more than some couples achieve in a lifetime, so give yourselves a pat on the back.

Day Seven
Kink: The Final Frontier

Welcome to the final day of *7 Days to Amazing Sex*. Just when you thought you knew everything there was to know about sex, I bring you here. Some of the sex acts explored today won't be to your taste, but I ask you to leave all your preconceptions at the door – not only because something you read might spark a desire in you, but also because if you pass judgement on something your partner secretly likes, they'll be less inclined to confide in you in the future.

So, I ask you to keep an open mind as we first take a closer look at group sex shenanigans, and then at the wild world of BDSM (bondage and discipline, domination and submission, and sadism and masochism), which I'll explain fully later.

You may feel inclined to incorporate a little kink into your love life from time to time, or you could discover it doesn't appeal to you, and that's fine. Today isn't about changing your sex life, it's about being armed with the knowledge to take things up a notch should you ever want to. As I always say, kink is great for a holiday, but I wouldn't want to live there. However, I also believe in the old adage, don't knock it till you've tried it (at least twice).

Exercise A

Is Three a Crowd? – Discover Whether Threesomes Are For You

Threesomes often come out top in surveys as the number-one sex fantasy most people would like to try out. But how do you know for sure whether you should make your fantasy a reality? This exercise is designed to reveal the answer and show you exactly what to do if you decide to go all the way.

The Yes Test

Before considering any kind of group sex, ask yourself which of the following statements apply to you, ringing 'Y' for yes and 'N' for no.

	Him	Her
I'm young and still exploring my sexuality; I crave sexual adventures and can separate sex and emotion.	Y / N	Y / N
I'm old enough to know what I want in bed and am beyond being coerced into anything against my better judgement.	Y / N	Y / N
I have high self-esteem.	Y / N	Y / N
I don't suffer with jealousy.	Y / N	Y / N
Jealousy is like an aphrodisiac for me.	Y / N	Y / N
I'm really bored with my sex life and have always fantasised about having group sex.	Y / N	Y / N
I think monogamy is unnatural.	Y / N	Y / N
I really want to sleep with other people but not behind my partner's back.	Y / N	Y / N
I think it would be a turn-on to watch my partner sleep with other people.	Y / N	Y / N
Ultimately, having group sex would be about sharing an intimate experience with my partner.	Y / N	Y / N

If *both* you and your partner said 'Yes' to five statements or more, then you may be ready to take the next step – that is, unless any of the following statements *also* apply to you:

- You suffer from feelings of jealousy.

- You suffer with insecurities about your body and low self-esteem.

- You feel you should try group sex because most of your friends have.

- You're only doing this because your partner wants to.

- You want to make your partner jealous, so you can see whether he/she really loves you.

The Fantasy Vs Reality Check

So, you think group sex is for you? Well, before you key 'Send me a swinger' into your Google search engine, let's take a moment to savour that orgiastic fantasy you must have been harbouring for a while now. I'm guessing it's perfect: you're the centre of attention, naturally, and you're orgasming so hard, you're surprised your feet don't blow right off.

But what if the reality is a little different? Or, what if it's a *lot* different?

Take a moment to replay your usual fantasy in your mind. Once you're 'in the zone', I'd like you to consider what your real-life reactions might be to the following possible scenarios:

- If the third party is the same sex as you and they undress, and you see that he has a much bigger penis / she has larger, perkier

> *Course Notes*
> ## Don't use kink as a mask
>
> Threesomes, foursomes and however many moresomes can destroy a relationship – particularly one that's using kinky sex as a way of masking or avoiding problems within the relationship. Don't enter into group sex without giving it a lot of thought, considering the negatives as well as the positives. The next part of this exercise is designed to make you do just that.

breasts than you, does that turn you on or make you feel less sexy by comparison?

- The third party and your partner become very involved with each other and there's no room for you to squeeze in for the time being. What do you do? How do you feel?

- Your partner has an orgasm with the third party – it's bigger and louder than the orgasms he/she usually has with you. Are you happy for them or worried that you don't satisfy your partner as much this third party seems able to do?

- You begin to have sex with the third party, but the chemistry's just not there. The moves that please your partner don't work for the third party, and you're beginning to lose your arousal. What do you do?

Real Sex
The Walk of Shame

I'd always liked the idea of a three-way and had a feeling that one day I'd try it. Then the opportunity came up after a party; everyone else had gone home, but the night still felt young (even though it was 3 a.m.) and my hosts – a couple I knew through a friend of a friend – invited me to stay on and have a few more drinks. Conversation turned to sex, then sex chat turned to drunken dares and I ended up kissing my female host, and it spiralled from there. At the time it seemed so cool and free-spirited, and, for a very short while, it was fun. But then I realised, I just couldn't come. The alcohol or the situation was holding me back, and when I knew I wasn't fully in the moment I quickly sobered up and wanted to leave. I went through the motions and gave the guy a blow-job, primarily because I didn't know how else to end it. Then I left feeling dirty. I still cringe at the thought of it now.

Alexis, 29

- You suddenly realise you're not turned on by the reality of group sex and that you much prefer the idea as a fantasy, but your partner is still really enjoying it. Do you: carry on? Stop? Ask you partner to stop? Or leave your partner to it?

● Then roles reverse: you're really enjoying yourself but you sense your partner is faking it, or that they feel vulnerable and upset just as you're close to climax. What do you do?

I don't mean to be a sex party pooper, and not all group sex experiences end in disappointment, but a *lot* of them do, and often because of the reasons above. To safeguard yourself against getting hurt (and hurting someone else) it's important to consider all possible outcomes and discuss them with your partner. When it comes to group sex, the only thing you can truly be sure of is that the reality will be nothing like the fantasy.

The Sex Party Planner

OK, you've considered the negatives, and have agreed that you're both prepared to take the risks involved in your quest for hedonistic sexual pleasure, so now it's time to plan the party. Read through the following pointers, then agree on who, where and what will feature in your first multiple hook-up. If you can't come to unanimous decisions, my advice would be to call the party off.

Who?

First up, how many people do you want to be involved in the session: three, four or more? If you're planning on a threesome you need to decide what gender the third party will be: male or female?

It's more common for women to be open to FFM (two females, one male) threesomes, than it is for men to want an MMF (two males, one female) configuration, because more women tend to more bicurious – or at least more women admit to it and are comfortable exploring it. In fact, that's the reason a lot of women suggest threesomes in the first place. However, same-sex individuals don't necessarily have to be physical with each other, so long as they're comfortable being naked together in the same room.

Generally, if you're a straight couple planning on a foursome, it works well to have another couple with an even number of men and women – with this configuration there's less chance of anyone feeling left out.

If you're going for a full-on orgy outside of your own home, gender is harder to control, and groups tend to be mixed (though in public venues, such as swingers' clubs, men often outnumber women – only slightly in good-quality establishments, more so in less sophisticated places).

The golden rule – and one that so many threesome-virgins break – is never to involve a friend. Should anything go wrong, your pal will serve as a constant reminder that you can't put behind you. You could develop feelings of jealousy or resentment towards them, and you could end up blaming them for it. And even if you don't feel that way, your friend might. It's far better to hire an escort from a reputable agency. A professional will know exactly what to do – it's just like the difference between getting a friend to fit a kitchen or a professional to do the job, you're likely to be much happier with the end result with the latter.

There's a saying that men don't pay prostitutes for the sex, they pay them to leave afterwards, and that's another bonus of using an escort service. While you should always be respectful and polite, you're buying the right to terminate the session whenever you please, without having to worry about how the third party feels; as long as they're treated decently and paid as agreed, an escort won't care if you simply couldn't go through with it. To them, you're just a job.

Extra-curricular Activity
Cam on

If you've met the object of your desires online, there's nothing to stop you from executing a 'dry run' with them in cyberspace before meeting in the flesh. This is a safe way to explore your group-sex fantasy without going all the way. Set up a webcam link to each other's computers and message each other with sexual instructions ('Push your fingers inside you'; 'Slide your tongue along his shaft' – that sort of thing). Afterwards, if you feel like you want more, you're a lot more likely to enjoy the reality; if, however, you feel a little disgusted with yourself, you can times that by ten to imagine how you'd feel after a real group session.

You can also find people to join a group session at organised soirées (see under 'Where?' on p. 177–8), or you can seek out a lover (or two, or three . . .) online. Type 'swingers' contacts' into a search engine for a list of options and then go people shopping.

All the usual safety rules apply to sharing information with strangers online: don't give out your real names, address or any other personal details that a stranger could identify you by. Get to know the person online first, and only then agree to meet in a safe, public place, like a bar in town (not your local pub!).

It's amazing how different a person (even one who's been completely honest and hasn't knocked five years off their age or ten inches off their waistline) can seem in real life. On meeting, you may decide there's no chemistry between you – this happens quite often among seasoned swingers, and there's no shame in admitting you don't feel a connection and moving on to the next person in your inbox.

If you do like the person/couple you've met, you can agree on a place to act out your fantasy – the question is: where?

Real Sex
The Swinging Professionals

My husband and I run a swingers' website and have been on the scene for years. We met our first couple online ourselves and drove several miles down the motorway to meet them – the meeting was meant as a 'get-to-know-you' rather than a 'get-into-bed-with-you', but we really clicked and the rest, as they say, is history.

While I really enjoy the exhibitionism, and my hubby really likes the sexual variety this lifestyle brings, for both of us, the sex we have together after being with another couple is what keeps us in the scene. It's like each swinging experience we share brings us closer together – like we're partners in crime or something. It revives our libidos (contrary to popular belief, not all swingers are nymphomaniacs), and it gives us something new to fantasise about. Despite running the site, we only actually indulge ourselves around three to four times a year, but that's just enough to keep things fresh between us. We do this because we want to stay together for ever, not because we want to be with other people.

Tilly, 36

Where?

Never meet strangers at your own home. The adapted adage 'Don't shag on your own doorstep' comes up a lot in swinging circles. For one, it's your home, so you can't leave if you want to. Secondly, it's downright dangerous to invite strangers into your home under any circumstances. Thirdly, what would you do if Aunt Hilda just happened to pop round?

Instead, arrange to meet at an organised (and reputable) swinging event. Some are thoroughly sleazy; others are glamorous events with strict entry codes – be prepared to be asked for photos of yourselves in advance, which will then be judged to determine whether you're attractive enough to be let in. Listings for all major events in your area will be posted online; just key 'swingers' events' into a search engine, and use your common sense to ascertain which parties are worth attending.

If you want total privacy, go to a hotel, or, better yet, book serviced apartments; these are apartments you can rent by the day, which are increasingly popular in the accommodation market. That way, you don't have to deal with a bemused receptionist booking three adults into one double room.

What?

With guests and venues sorted, all that remains is for you to lay some plans and ground rules, first as a couple, then with the lovers who'll be sharing your bed. So, are you happy for your partner to kiss the third party, but don't want them to have penetrative sex with them? Or, are you fine with penetrative sex, but view kissing as something intimate, only to be shared between you and your other half? And what about the third (fourth, etc. ...) person – do they want to be kissed, or is that off-limits? Is oral sex on the menu or off?

Discussing all these details beforehand may seem like a blow to spontaneity, but you can take the

Course Notes
One for the ride

Avoid drinking too much alcohol (and taking any other mind-altering substances), as it really is important to keep a clear head when experimenting with group sex. For the record, anything beyond one glass is too much. If you have to get drunk (or high) in order to go through with group sex, that's your subconscious telling you that it is not something you really want to do. Also, alcohol numbs the genitals, so it's a total waste of your time, and while under the influence of booze, you may think you're the best thing that's ever happened to sex, but in reality your bedfellows will see you as a drunk with poor hand-to-eye co-ordination who can't quite hit the spot. Hopefully that image will be enough to put you off that second Shiraz!

conversation to a flirty, tactile level over a glass of wine (*just the one! –* see Course Notes opposite); arming yourselves with these details now will prevent any *really* awkward, mood-killing moments later on.

It should go without saying that safe sex is crucial, but just in case: SAFE SEX IS CRUCIAL. Have an industrial supply of condoms at the ready; every time a man changes partners he needs to change his condom; every time a toy is used to penetrate a different orifice, it needs a change of condom. You should also consider using latex gloves (for manual stimulation) and latex squares to cover genitals (for oral stimulation) as some infections can be spread via mouths and fingers. Both latex gloves and squares are available online, and in some pharmacies (latex squares are also sometimes referred to as dental dams).

Extra-curricular Activity
Watch and learn

Without committing to get involved in anything, go to a swingers' party as voyeurs. Don't worry; this is perfectly acceptable practice on the scene. A lot of participants go precisely because they're aroused by their own exhibitionism.

Watching real-life group-sex sessions (rather than those you see in porn films) is the best way to learn what to expect and how to execute sex with multiple partners. At the same time, witnessing the realities will help you to know for sure whether it's what you really want. If you come away feeling angry because your partner was getting turned on by watching another man or woman, you can guess at just how bad you would feel if they had actually been having sex with them.

Finally, so you don't get lost in action, it pays to have a few ideas up your foreskin (I'm guessing sleeves will be non-existent by this point). There are a few classic multiple-partner configurations that are popular enough to have earned monikers. First there's 'DP', which simply stands for double penetration, applied in MMF threesomes where one man penetrates a woman vaginally while another penetrates her anally. Then there's the depictive 'spit roast' – call me a prude, but I hate that term – where a woman has penetrative sex with one man while giving another oral sex. I assume it feels better than it sounds. There's also the altogether more pleasant-sounding 'daisy chain' in which every partner present is linked to another via mouth, hands or genitals, forming a complete circle. So, woman A could be giving oral sex to man B, who is also going down on woman C, who is masturbating man D, who is giving oral sex to woman A – and so the chain is complete. (Tip: if you find 69s too complicated, this last move isn't the one for you.)

A simpler strategy is what I call the 2–4–1 formation. Two people focus all their attention on one person at a time. This marries up to most people's fantasy of what a threesome will be like for them – at least for a third of the time at any rate, assuming you all play fair.

Exercise B

What Does BDSM Stand For, Anyway? – A Beginner's Guide to Power Play

BDSM is an overlapping acronym that represents the following:

Bondage – using restraints such as rope, chains and cuffs on a partner.

Discipline – training and disciplining a submissive partner using bondage, physical punishment, such as caning and verbal reprimands.

Domination – controlling a submissive partner using all the above methods.

Submission – relinquishing all control to a dominant partner.

Sadism – pleasure from inflicting pain on others.

Masochism – pleasure from receiving pain from others.

While some lovers take BDSM to the extreme, many others have taken part without even realising it. Ever played with fluffy handcuffs, slapped a lover's behind, or pinned your partner's arms down during lovemaking? All these things fall into the mild end of the BDSM spectrum.

In fact power play is present in just about all sexual relationships. Do you always initiate sex, but your partner actually controls whether or not you have sex? Do you find you're more passive in bed, while you partner is more likely to suggest or request certain acts? This is power play at work, and learning to harness it can make for some interesting times between the sheets.

In this exercise, we're going to take a closer look at this complex form of role play based on the exchange of power, so you can decide if you want to utilise it to spice up your sex life.

Real Sex
A Slave to Love

I love to surrender myself to my partner – and I surrender all of myself: the personas I adopt as mum, wife, employee, all my worries and concerns – I leave everything at the bedroom door, and all that's left of me is my sexual self, ready to serve. It gives me a natural high and acts as my weekly stress relief. I couldn't live without those sessions. Friends who know – friends who aren't part of the BDSM scene – think it's bizarre, but it's a ritual pleasure for me. I like the feeling of bondage tape pressing down on my breasts, of my legs being forced open so my master can inspect between my legs, of his member pushing into my mouth. And the blindfold keeps me guessing about whether I'll receive a warm, wet lick with a tongue or a harsh lick of the whip. It doesn't hurt – all I feel is adrenalin and, finally, when I'm allowed sex, the best orgasms ever.

Juliet, 29

What's Your Sexual Style?

With BDSM, the first thing to consider is whether you'd like to play the dominant or submissive role, otherwise known as the dom/'top'/master or mistress or the sub/'bottom'/slave, respectively. Of course, you don't always have to be one or the other. Most people have both submissive and dominant aspects to their personalities, so feel free to switch (but not during the same session – that would just mess with the ambience).

You might like occasionally to adopt a submissive role if:

- You want to relinquish responsibility in the bedroom as a form of escapism because your life or your job already involves enough of this.

- You want to relinquish emotional responsibility because you feel the sex you crave is somehow wrong or taboo, but when another person is 'forcing' you to do it, it's not your fault and you're therefore free to enjoy it more (this could work well, for example, for men who want to be anally penetrated by their partners, but can't get over the association with homosexuality; if his mistress is 'forcing' him to take it, her desires rather than his are to blame).

- You want to relinquish all control because you like to be the centre of attention and have everything done for (or to) you; but at the same time you can take on the role of serving your master or mistress, trusting and following their instructions.

- You get turned on by the idea of being treated like a sex object and called taboo names like 'slut' or 'scum'.

You might like to try your hand at bedroom domination if:

- Your partner always initiates sex and you want to take control for a change.

- You like the idea of being able to order your partner to satisfy you in any way that you desire (this is certainly one way to make sex instruction kinky rather than clinical!).

- You like the idea of being able to tease your partner mercilessly.

- You get turned on by being in control in sexual situations and have a good sexual imagination that can conjure up interesting scenarios for both yourself and your sub to enjoy (but don't be fooled: there's more to being a dom than saying, 'Hey you, give me a blow-job, now!', or, 'Slave, get in that kitchen and wash the dishes' – if that were the case there wouldn't be a non-practising man or woman in the land; playing dom is actually hard work, and while you can demand those things, you need to keep your sub entertained at all times and that requires intuition and cunning and the right mix of punishment and reward).

- you're aroused by using traditionally offensive, taboo language in a sexual setting and like the idea of verbally degrading someone for their (and your) sexual pleasure.

Real Sex
Bedroom Domination

I adore women, and taking control in a positive and erotic situation comes naturally to me. It's a delicious exchange between two people who have different but complementary needs.

Taking a woman to the place where she gives herself to you completely is a gorgeous experience and a powerful thrill, and it happens because the focus is on her and her needs. The place she can go to in her head is one where she can be pure woman: an object of desire and passion. As well as the physical pleasure, there's the spiritual connection of sharing that unique time together.

The submission can often include a degree of controlled pain, and that can be hugely liberating and erotic. It breaks psychological barriers down, releases endorphins, and requires a degree of trust in my control that can become a dizzying sexual rush. That trust means I have a responsibility of care, and I enjoy that.

Greg, 45

But you should *never* play with BDSM if:

- You view it as a way to vent real anger or punish a lover for unresolved issues within your relationship; BDSM play is a form of safe and consensual role play, *not* an opportunity for revenge.
- You view it as a way to abuse yourself or reinforce low self-esteem or abusive behaviour you've experienced in the past.
- You're under the influence of alcohol or illegal or prescription drugs – drink and drugs can numb the senses, making any sex play that involves even a small amount of pain or binding of body parts extremely dangerous; you need to be able to feel your

pain threshold clearly, so you can make informed decisions as to whether you'd like to cross that threshold and by how much.

● You haven't researched the basic BDSM safety rules; read on to get acquainted, before even thinking about going any further.

The rules of BDSM

Rule # 1. The first rule of BDSM is to know your safe words (or signals). This is essential because BDSM is the one area of sex where 'No' doesn't always mean no – but that's *only* when it's agreed prior to play that protestations will be part of the game. So the sub can scream, 'No, stop, please, no . . . ' when really they're thinking, 'Yes, please, more, more, more'. In order to do this safely, both players agree a code in which, for example, 'red' means stop, 'amber' means bring it down a notch and 'green' means more intensity, please! If a verbal code isn't plausible (if you have a ball gag in your mouth, for instance), then agree a sign-language code that can be clearly read, such as holding two fingers in the air.

Rule # 2. When binding someone, be careful not to restrict blood flow. As a general rule, any binding you create should be loose enough for you to get your finger beneath it. If it isn't, loosen it, and continually check bindings, as movement, such as struggling during play, can cause binds to tighten further. Keys and scissors should always be within easy reach to free your sub quickly if you need to. And, finally, whoever is bound, should use their safe word if they feel any numbness, cramping or pins and needles in their body at any time.

Rule # 3. Spanking and whipping should be done with extreme care. Never strike the lower back (the kidneys are close to the surface and easily damaged) and direct your aim to the fleshier parts of the body, such as buttocks and thighs.

Rule # 4. Remove contact lenses before applying a blindfold, as pressure on the eyes while wearing contacts can cause damage.

Rule # 5. All the usual rules of safe sex also apply, such as using condoms on penises and toys to prevent the spread of STIs and using lubricant for anal sex. There is good pain, which is controllable, temporary and releases endorphins, and then there's bad pain, which can cause permanent damage – tearing the delicate anal tissue is definitely the latter. Also, I would never recommend anyone take BDSM this far, but extreme whipping can break the skin, and, as such, all flogging tools should be sanitised.

Real Sex
A Question of Character

I have been a professional dominatrix for over four years and a part of the BDSM scene for many more. The key to making this sort of role play really get inside your head and free you of all your inhibitions is to stay in character at all times during a session. It's no use saying, 'Honey, can we take a quick break? I need to pee', when you're trying to play submissive. You need to say, 'Master [or Mistress], please may I be excused to go to the bathroom?' and accept their decision, whatever it is, even if that means wetting the bed. Nine out of ten times a dom isn't going to push their sub that far unless that's what they believe the sub wants, but it's crucial a dom has that control. The further you're prepared to go, the better it will get, and so long as you have a safe word, you're never going to get hurt.

Mistress A., 35

Tools of the Trade

BDSM is a sport that requires props – and those props are what will help get you into character. So, if you've decided you want to experiment, scout around your home for suitable apparatus or go shopping for something a little more *un*comfortable to slip into. Here's the line-up of what could give your vanilla-sex sessions a kinky flavour, plus my suggested household alternatives.

- **Outfits.** The gothic and rubber attire of the BDSM scene may not be rocking this season's catwalks, but there's something to be said (particularly for women) for zipping yourself into a tight little rubber number. The restrictive fabric helps to sculpt your body and forces you to stand tall, making it perfect for channelling your dominant side.

    A friend of mine is a professional dominatrix and, while looking at her holiday snaps recently, I realised that she even wears restrictive PVC rubber bikinis on the beach! For my friend, the right clothes create the right attitude, and when she's with a slave, she's in costume 24/7 to manifest her sexual powers.

Unfortunately, this sort of clobber also tends to be very expensive, so why not improvise with what you have at home? Ladies can't go wrong with black lingerie, red lips and nails and stacked black stilettos – it's a classic cliché, but it works. Gents should wear something they're comfortable in, but that's also sexy; if you feel like an idiot in black leather pants you will look like one, but make no effort at all and your lack of commitment to your career will ensure it never gets off the ground. Maybe just jeans, plain black karate-style pyjama bottoms or a robe would work.

For a sub-style outfit, try customising underwear by cutting out the crotch to expose the genitals; and the same trick can work with a bra. Or try a simple dog collar with matching frilly knickers for her – or even for him!

● **Restraints.** There's a confusing array of equipment designed to bind arms, legs and torsos, including bondage belts featuring hoops that act as anchoring points for other restraints, such as wrist cuffs, and spreader bars – solid rods that attach to ankle cuffs to keep legs forced apart. For bondage beginners it's far better to keep things simple.

In high-street sex stores the most popular items sold are basic handcuffs and bondage tape. Handcuffs are great for bad cop role-play scenarios, and though they may look a little twee covered in faux fur, a fabric cover prevents the metal from digging into your flesh. The worst thing about traditional handcuffs is that they require keys; most sets come with a spare, so store both keys separately in safe places, otherwise you may find yourself calling on the fire services with a rather embarrassing request.

Bondage tape looks like a roll of PVC carpet tape and comes in sexy shades, including black, red and hot pink; you can even get tape covered with rose and heart tattoo designs. Unlike carpet tape, this stuff doesn't stick to your skin, but rather to itself, and can be rolled back up after play and used again. It's amazing stuff – I've even seen female celebs *wear* it as an outfit, wrapped several times around themselves.

A household alternative to bondage tape is cling film (though I wouldn't be seen wearing that around town). It's more fiddly than bondage tape when it comes to binding wrists or ankles, but it's great for wrapping all around a lover's torso, pinning their arms to their sides, rendering them helpless. As a bonus, the tension caused by the film can heighten sensation in the skin – try blowing on it, licking your partner through it, or trailing an ice cube across it to tease your lover's senses. When you're done, you can carefully snip it off.

In place of cuffs, you can use silk scarves, ties or stockings and bind ankles or wrists together, but think first about the positions you'll be putting your lover into. For example, it would be better to bind ankles individually to bed posts or chair legs if you will need your lover's legs to be open later. Also, when making knots that could take time to undo, it's essential to keep scissors handy so you can cut through any binds in a hurry if necessary.

Real Sex
Hanky Spanky

I would never want to be whipped – I'm not into pain at all, but dishing it out is a different matter. I like to dress up like a city chick or a dominatrix and take control of my boyfriend. I have him strip naked and kneel on all fours with his bum pointing towards me. I alternate my spanks or whips on his cheeks and leave different durations between them. So, I might do five quick, soft ones in a row, then a big hard one and then wait a whole minute before another one, so he never knows when the next blow will come. Also, I've noticed if I cup my hand when spanking, the sound is better and louder. Afterwards, I gently blow on the sore areas, lick them with the tip of my tongue and run my palm over them. He tells me he's really sensitive to my hands by the time I do this, so it's like the ultimate caress.

Ashlie, 24

● **Whips, floggers, crops, canes and paddles.** The range of whipping and spanking devices has surprising diversity.

Floggers are whips with several, short (usually leather) fronds at the end, most commonly nine in total (hence the moniker 'cat-o'-nine-tails'). They're easier to handle, as they strike a wider area and are less likely to cause damage, but should still be wielded with care. Novelty versions, like the one I have with so many thin, soft, rubber fronds at the end that it looks like a cheerleader's pompom, can be gently whipped across the skin for a little sting 'n' tingle without causing any harm, then gently stroked back over the same stretch of skin to soothe.

Note: don't even think about using a long single-tail whip (also known as a 'bullwhip', the sort used to handle livestock, which make a cracking sound in the air) – you need to be specially trained for that. Canes and crops have been used to belt people for years, and older readers may already have had the pleasure/pain (depending on your persuasion) at the hands of parents and teachers before such punishments were outlawed.

Paddles are seen as entry-level spanking devices, though many couples never feel the need to go any further, their dalliance with BDSM beginning and ending here. Paddles are probably so popular because they're the safest and easiest of all spanking apparatus to use and they're arguably just as much fun. Used on the fleshiest part of the butt, a paddle sends vibrations through the genitals and leaves a warm mild sting on the cheeks. Some paddles have leather or rubber on one side (for smacking with) and faux fur or velvet on the other (for alternating with soft strokes). You can even get paddles featuring raised heart shapes in the centre, to leave cute imprints on your lover's flesh.

For household alternatives, try a ping-pong paddle, a large wooden spoon, a small chopping board with a handle, a flat plastic spatula or even a slipper.

● **Blindfolds and gags.** You can buy blindfolds from sex shops, lingerie boutiques and even health and beauty stores; my favourite blindfold (faux black satin with red velvet lining) came free in a passenger pack on a long-haul Virgin flight. Or you can improvise with any length of fabric in the home.

Blindfolding a partner will increase their anticipation levels and heighten their other senses, but some people really get off on the view and won't appreciate being deprived of it, no matter how magnified their sense of touch becomes. Think about that (and how much effort you've made with your look) before deciding whether to get your blindfold out.

Likewise, gags eliminate a person's ability to join in on any sexy pillow talk.

You might remember seeing Bruce Willis waking up in a ball gag in *Pulp Fiction*. These balls, attached to head harnesses, act as a stopper in the mouth. They're uncomfortable to wear and they inhibit communication, plus they make you drool (never a good look) – so, for all these reasons, I'd avoid this type of gag completely. If you want to role play 'capture and kidnap' scenarios as part of a BDSM session, wrap a stocking across the mouth, or better yet, ball up some skimpy knickers (unworn or worn, whatever your preference as the dom) and use those instead. But make sure breathing isn't hampered in any way, and remember to agree on a safe word in sign language that means, 'OK, get these pants out of my mouth now', before you start.

Real Sex
Bad Girl

69

I always thought spanking was a bit contrived but that all changed when my fiancé and I were play-fighting one day and he dragged me over his knee then gave me a hard spanking. Suddenly, it really turned me on – something about the submissive nature of it, and being punished for being 'naughty' and fighting him was fun. Now it's a regular part of our sex life. He's a master of starting slowly and gradually ramping it up; and he'll often pull his hand back hard, then only spank lightly, so I don't know whether to tense up or relax – it's a good mind-game. Oddly, the idea of spanking him just makes me laugh – but giving him a passionate movie-style slap round the face can be hot!

Lucy, 32

Candles. Dripping molten candle wax on to your lover's bare flesh can sensitise their skin without burning it – *if* it's done carefully with the right type of candle. Of course, candles *are* household items, but I don't recommend using anything that's coloured or scented or made from beeswax, as these all burn at too high a temperature. Plain white paraffin candles are the only ones you can get away with and here's a hot (or rather cooling) tip: the greater the height you drip the wax from, the cooler it will be when it lands on the skin, so keep your candle at least 40–50cm away from the skin. Blow out the candle before you start dripping, and when the wax lands, rub it across your partner's skin to disperse the heat. Also, when pouring wax, take great care to avoid splashes on your furniture and sheets – wax is murder to get out of upholstery and fabrics. If you need to, though, scrape away excess wax, then place paper towels over the stain and then go over it with an iron – the wax re-melts and is absorbed by the paper.

An easier, safer option is to invest in a purpose-made massage candle. The wax melts into a body oil and the containers have lips so you can them pour the warm oil over your partner. Follow with an ice cube for intense hot 'n' cold thrills that will make your lover's nerve endings stand to attention.

Real Sex
Wax Works

I remember the night my boyfriend introduced me to candle wax. He used a special candle that melts at a lower temperature, so it's not searing on your skin, and it can be massaged in afterwards. He dripped the wax from a height on my breasts and stomach – it was very theatrical. The first touch was shockingly hot, but not exactly painful – just unexpected. Then he rubbed it into my skin and it smelt wonderful. Another time, he had me blindfolded and bent over on my front, then he dripped a trail of wax down my back and on to my bottom. The blindfold meant that I was uber-sensitive to the wax and gave me this real sense of trusting my partner, even though I knew I wasn't at any risk.

Emma, 30

● **Nipple clamps.** These alligator-style clips are usually made from metal but the tips are coated in soft rubber (or at least they should be!) to protect the delicate skin of the nipples. The clamps may be connected to each other via a chain so they can be tugged in unison, or they may be connected to a vibrating unit for added buzz. Some are adjustable so you can tighten the clamps' grip as the wearer becomes used to the sensation (or misbehaves). Time spent playing with circulation in this way should never exceed ten minutes, so make sure you keep an eye on that bedroom clock!

The reason clamps are so popular is because the nipples are major erogenous zones, and reducing circulation in them increases their sensitivity even further. In fact, if you have little or no sensation in your nipples, using clamps will actually develop responsiveness here for you.

Not ready to invest in your first set of nipple clamps? Well, they may not be as sexy to look at, but household clothes pegs do just as good a job for beginners, and while you can't adjust them as you could a swanky tailor-made pair, you can pinch less skin for higher intensity and more skin between them for lower intensity.

But be warned, the highest level of pain comes when you take the clamps off rather than when you put them on, so try a few one-minute trials to see how you react before going for a full-on session.

Being happy with your sex life is not always about acting on your desires; sometimes it's just about understanding them. The last day of my plan should have answered a lot of questions about some of your darker desires, as well as giving you some alternative ideas for those times when you feel like giving your sex life a more drastic shake-up (even if it's just for one night).

I'd also like to point out that, if I'd written this book a few years ago, strap-on dildos being used on straight men would have featured in the kink section, rather than in Day Five, among standard sex toys. While using anal toys on men in heterosexual relationships is still relatively new and uncommon, what was once firmly in the domain of the BDSM scene has crossed into the mainstream market where these toys are now being sold. Over time, anally pleasuring straight men will become less taboo until, eventually, it'll be seen as just another thing that couples do (in much the same way that using female sex toys eventually lost its forbidden status). My point is that what seems wild today will probably seem 'normal' tomorrow, so always be governed by what makes *you and your partner* feel sexy, rather than by what you think is socially acceptable. If you do that, and stay true to your heart and loins, your sex life will always be a thrill.

Graduation

Before you embarked on my plan and pledged to follow *7 Days to Amazing Sex*, I told you about a special treatment that could make you look and feel younger and tone up in all the right places. I told you how science had proven that the same treatment could act as a cure for insomnia and headaches and even defend against more serious conditions, and that the same treatment would boost your self-esteem and improve your relationship.

You now know that this 'miracle' treatment is sex, and if you've followed my seven-day plan you should already be feeling the benefits. But this is just the beginning.

To graduate with honours from my programme and reap *all* its rewards to the full, you must commit to incorporating everything you've learnt into your day-to-day life from this moment on. That means:

- Making time to indulge in solo sex – pampering, exploring and, most importantly, appreciating your amazing body, while allowing your partner the space and trust to do the same.

- Bringing variety to your sex life by using your hands and mouth in artful ways and remembering that lovemaking isn't restricted to penetrative sex – in fact, it doesn't even necessarily need to be included at all (sometimes, absence makes the loins grow fonder!).

- Being playful and inventive, and brave enough to suggest new positions, techniques or toys – as well as appreciating that time spent considering new ideas for the bedroom is a great libido booster and foreplay for you in itself.

● Continually communicating with your partner, from sharing fantasies to more serious chats about any sexual issues you may have, because the more fluent you become in all forms of sex talk, the happier (and hotter) your relationship will be.

If, at this stage, you feel you still need to work on developing your sex skills in a certain area – for example, oral sex – simply go back and repeat the relevant day of the programme. And if, in the future, your sex life is starting to flag, go through the programme again, fitting it around your schedule or taking it away on holiday for a solid week of sexy relationship therapy. With *7 Days to Amazing Sex* at your side, you need never have a lacklustre love life again.

So, congratulations on graduating, and welcome to your future – one that is paved with good health, pleasure and endless sexual adventures.

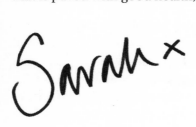

Resources

Erotica

Cliterati.co.uk

Amateur authors share their written erotica, while all visitors to the site are invited to upload their own.

ScarletMagazine.co.uk

Signing up for free membership allows site visitors to download free erotic stories from the magazine's *Cliterature* supplement.

StrictlyBroadband.co.uk

A fabulous site featuring all the latest celebrity sex-scandal tapes, as well as a mind-blowing selection of adult films covering all genres, plus categories specifically for women and couples, all downloadable for a small fee.

YouPorn.com

A free adult site featuring an amazing array of amateur videos to suit all tastes. Exhibitionists can upload their own contributions.

Group Sex and Swinging

AdultFriendFinder.com

This is the world's biggest site for swingers and group-sex enthusiasts, where you can find a third party or couple to join you for fun. Simply key in what you're looking for (man, woman, couple), then sign up for free membership and start window-shopping.

FeverParties.com

With a first-timers' guide, this site is dedicated to swinging parties for the young and attractive only; you must apply to attend a party by sending in a picture of yourself. Some believe this is too exclusive, while others find it reassuring. Older guests (aged thirty to fifty) should follow the link to Fervour parties. Events tend to be London-based, but there are occasional parties outside of the capital.

Swing2Us.com

Long-standing UK-based contact site for couples looking for couples, with useful features such as swinging holiday listings, chat rooms, advice on swinging and links to other reputable swinging sites.

Sex Toy Retailers

AnnSummers.com

This site features a store locator service for the UK's leading high-street sex toy retailer, so you can find a branch near you. Alternatively, shop online for sex toys, lingerie and adult novelties.

Babeland.com

This brilliant site is linked to the Babeland store, first opened by Claire Cavanah and Rachel Venning in 1993 in response to the lack of women-friendly sex shops in Seattle, US. Since then two more stores have opened in New York and Los Angeles. All stores offer a programme of events including sex talks and workshops, which are listed on the site, along with their wide range of sex toys and accessories. You can also order by calling (+001) 800 658 9119.

GoodVibes.com

The San Francisco-based retailer Good Vibrations became big news when it was set up in 1977 to offer women a safe environment in which to shop for sex toys. Ever since it's been providing women with sound advice and sex aids through it's web site and growing chain of stores. It also sells toys for boys and safe sex essentials including condoms, dams and gloves.

Lovehoney.co.uk

One of the best sex toy sites in the UK by far, selling all the latest and most innovative products and sex accessories such as hot wax massage candles and sex furniture; it also features video demonstrations showing how toys work, a toy recycling service and a free sex toy magazine – ideal for novices and aficionados alike. Plus, there's a 24-hour order line: 0800 915 6635.

Onjoy.com

Beautiful online boutique selling a huge range of sex toys and accessories, categorised by toys 'for him', 'for her', 'for couples' and 'lingerie', making it a well-presented site that's easy to navigate. Call 0800 310 1323 for their free 24-hour order line.

RealDoll.com

The original lifelike sex doll retailer offers a bespoke service, allowing customers to create their ideal silicone partner.

SexToys.co.uk

This is the UK's leading discount toy store for adults, making it an ideal choice for shoppers on a budget. Prices are low and the quality of service is high, and there are hundreds of gadgets to choose from.

BritishCondoms.co.uk

If you like variety when it comes to safe sex, this site is the one for you, stocking everything from dental dams to glow-in-the-dark condoms. Call 0845 600 8256.

Dressing Up

AgentProvocateur.com

Luxury lingerie boutique Agent Provocateur has earned a name for itself as the sexiest high-end purveyor of intimates in the world, with famously decadent stores as far and wide as Russia, Asia and the Middle East. As well as selling the sort of lingerie that makes role-play feel sexy rather than silly, Agent Provocateur offers a selection of accessories including designer blindfolds and whips and paddles, and everything is designed with one goal in mind: 'to give you the confidence to give in to your deepest desires.' Shop online, or visit their site to find your nearest boutique.

Sex Therapy

Counsel-search.com

US-based readers can find the closest marriage counselors and therapists in their state using this simple search site; there's also a section addressing frequently asked questions regarding marriage counselling.

Relate.org.uk

Relate offers advice, relationship counselling, sex therapy, workshops, mediation, consultations and support face-to-face, by phone and through its website. To find your nearest Relate centre, call 0300 100 1234.

Sexual Health

CDC.gov/sexualhealth

This US Government site provides advice and the latest reports on all sexual health issues from the prevention of sexual violence to HIV testing. US residents can call free on (+001) 800 232 4636.

CondomEssentialWear.co.uk

This NHS-backed site provides tips on how to make condoms a fun and essential part of your sex life, plus useful information about STIs. You can also call the confidential sexual health helpline on 0800 567 123 with any specific questions.

DurexWorld.com

As well as selling the most innovative range of safe-sex products from flavoured condoms and tingling, sex-enhancing lubricants to penis rings and vibrators, this site provides essential information on STIs and sex in general.

NHS.uk

The UK's National Health Service site contains clear and accurate information about sexual health, STIs, symptoms and cures. You can also call NHS Direct to speak to a trained nurse to talk through any concerns you have on 0845 4647.

Index

sex
by numbers
SARAH HEDLEY

Everything you need to know about
sex and a few things you shouldn't

Sex by Numbers is packed with fascinating facts and lists which answer every question you have about sex. From the most potent sexual positions and best ever oral techniques to the top ten classic parody porn titles, this light-hearted but essential guide includes everything you have ever wondered about:

- **The body** – a guide to erogenous zones, massage, masturbation and sexual positions

- **Sexual accessories** – including sex toys, orgasm-boosting condoms and household objects to help you climax

- **Games for grown-ups** – including outdoor fun, fantasies and bondage

- **Food of lust** – foolproof recipes to boost your libido and the aphrodisiacs you should avoid

- **Sex on screen** – from introducing your partner to porn to finding the sexiest bonkbusters ever

Sex by Numbers will expand your knowledge beyond the realms of decency, and even necessity, guaranteeing that you'll always be both satisfied and satisfying between the sheets – not to mention full of hot trivia at dinner parties.

ISBN: 978 0 7499 2696 1